1. Every Woman's Face is her Glory.

2. We don't want to be Well Preserved.

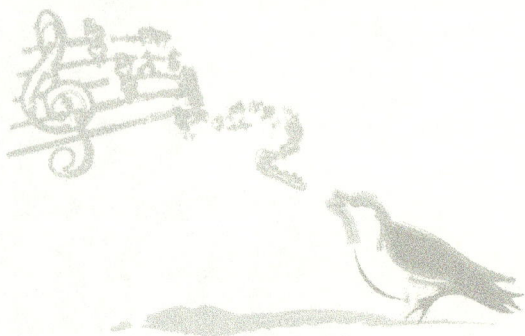

Contents

Contents

978-1-4457-1477-6

978-1-4457-1477-6

Acknowledgements

Many thanks are due to Tallulah and Nadia Annette, the human guinea pigs who tried out all exercises and reported difficult or ambigious parts of the instructions. Sean and Lois Martin and Lu Milne for their support, to Claire and Sabel who took the photographs, to all the girls (and the occasional guy) on the Ageless forum for their encouragement, for reporting their progress, and for helping me realise where I needed to explain better.

Michael Ward, who designed this edition, and the cover, gets special thanks for his hard work, patience, and for making the book look so lovely.

My lovely friend and coach Anne Waldon is teaching me

to become incomparable. She can teach you too:

Riverdragoncoaching.co.uk

Note: People have commented on how different my nose and jaw look in the pics of me in my thirties. The shape of my nose was altered in January 2009, when I had surgery to correct a deviated septum and straighten out my nose.

So here are a couple of pictures of me before I had the operation. My nose photographs very differently at different angles as it was extremely crooked, but in both these pictures I've had no facial surgery. I've never had anything done to my jaw, the difference you see is simply the way I naturally hold the jaw now, rather than allowing it to drop forward.

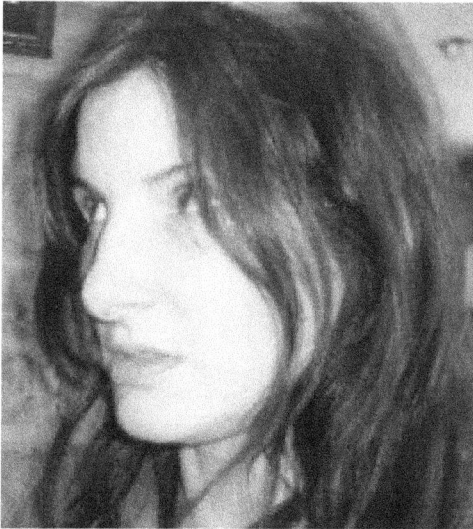

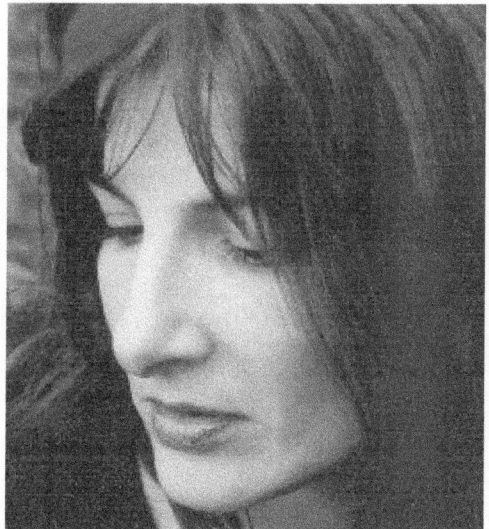

Dedicated to
Pat Pickering

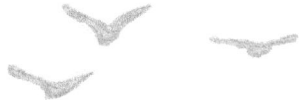

Fame at last

*also love to
baby Freya*

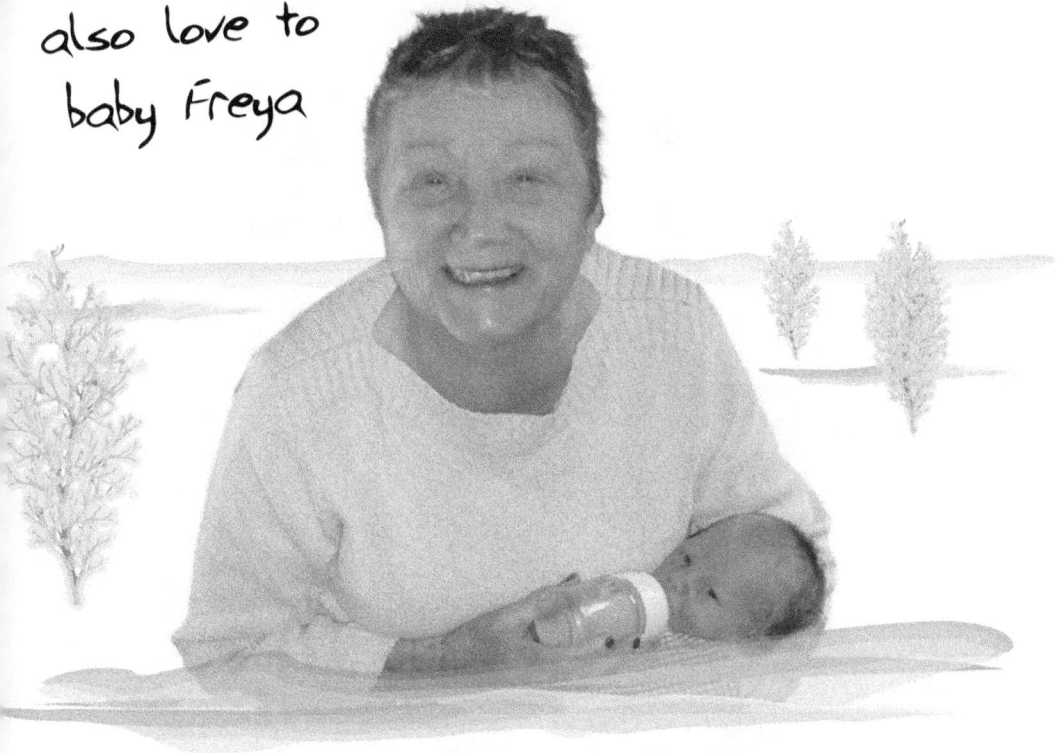

Physically, a man is a man for a much longer time
than a woman is a woman.

~Honoré de Balzac, *The Physiology of Marriage*

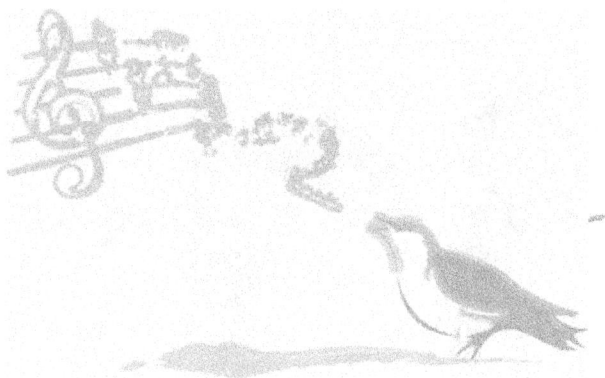

Chapter one
Some encouragement

How to treat real skin

Nobody questions that facial skin is extremely delicate, to be touched gently and rarely, and preferably by a professional. We don't trust our own hands near the face and don't use them for anything more daring than applying a serum.

The facial skin has moved into a separate category from the organ that covers the rest of the body. It's not only super-delicate, it's often not living at all. It's canvas to put make-up on--dead, to all intents and purposes, so that mistakes are forever, and the consequences of doing something unexpected to it don't bear thinking about. No wonder we feel vulnerable and need the expertise of large companies to formulate skin care and guide product choices.

We grew up with the image of the skin as a canvas for eye shadow and blusher, and from there we've somehow got the idea that it really is a canvas, a very fragile one that is always on the brink of falling to pieces. We accept the idea of older women being 'well preserved', as though we're aiming, with an increasing lack of success, to recreate the face we had at 20 by means of applying moisturiser, as if the skin were a leather sofa.

It's convenient to think like this, because the layer that over-the-counter products and salon facials have most effect on is dead, ready to be rubbed away over the following days or weeks.

9

A moisturiser or a rejuvenating product will improve the appearance of this top layer of cells, but it can't do much at all for the deeper layers that affect how we'll look long-term. If a product could affect the function of the skin and have a significant effect on existing damage it would be a drug, like the prescription-only tretinoin (Retin-A).

And we accept the assumption that facial skin can be pulled out of shape and rendered unwearable like a woollen jumper. No it can't, because it's nothing like a woollen jumper. It behaves like other organs of the body, heart, lungs, and skeletal muscles, and it adapts to being exercised by growing stronger, or on the other hand, it responds to lack of stimulation and challenge with a decline in strength and resilience.

It's not easy to have faith in the skin when everyone feels they know with absolute certainty that you should never drag or stretch it. But the skin loves being stretched. It feels really good, just like stretching the muscles feels good in bed or at a yoga session. Nobody suggests that stretching the muscles will pull them out of shape... elasticity is the ability of the tissue to regain its original shape, not a dangerous business that causes the limbs to come loose.

Once you start to handle your skin with conviction you'll feel it coming to life under your hands, and you'll be delighted that you trusted yourself to reconnect with your own face rather than allowing the skin to lie inert and untouchable. At the same time you have the skin thickening and growing more elastic over the days and weeks.

Lifting up the face

There's so much hope resting on the rejuvenation of the skin, and yet the condition of the skin has a relatively small effect on the appearance of the face. We think, broadly, of firming and tightening the skin and using it to hold the muscular structure of the face in place, as if that was the function our skin performed when we were young. It's entirely back-to-front thinking.

On the rest of the body, where the skin forms a separate layer that just wraps a limb or a shoulder without attachment to the muscle, the tone of the skin is independent of muscle tone. The skin on the stomach isn't joined to the abdominal muscles anywhere. Doing sit-ups won't tighten the skin there, and it is very annoying for people who have given birth that so many people believe it will.

The muscles that express emotion... raise the eyebrows, crinkle the eyes, and smile... are attached to the skin that they move around to form these expressions. Facial skin tissue and muscle fibres flow into each other in many parts of a face. Restoring tone in the facial muscles will naturally lift the skin and draw it towards the bone structure. It's perverse to firm the face by surgically tightening the skin. The skin doesn't hold the muscle in place... the muscle holds the skin in place. Given that this is the case, it makes infinitely more sense to work on the muscle than on the skin. We will do both.

Cause and treatment of facial wrinkling

The reason for wrinkling is obvious once you realise it has nothing to do with creasing the skin as such.

Wrinkle formation seems a very technical business involving many discussions of cells and blood and dissections of the skin, but all that is besides the point, and how wrinkles form is very easy to understand.

Making an expression will leave wrinkles, but it's not a case of thin delicate skin being crushed like a tissue. When you make a face, you're moving a thick chunk of flesh (skin and muscle fused together), like a tablecloth with a thick backing, and the wrinkles form in the same way, as they'd form if the backing was pulled out of shape.... Say it shrank in the wash and the upper fabric didn't, or some of the threads caught and bunched up areas of the backing fabric or even if you pulled at one corner of the backing fabric, the upper layer would wrinkle. If you managed to get the backing layer straight again, say you stop pulling and the backing layer lies flat there might be some residual creases, but the deep, furrowy wrinkles will disappear.

11

Another way to understand this is to imagine a piece of fabric made into a tight-fitting mask and bonded to your face.... It would wrinkle as the face moved. But if you put the mask on so that it was only glued at the edges it would wrinkle much less as the fabric can distribute the distortion along its whole length and width. You can see, then, that the attachment of facial muscles to the skin is necessary for the formation of deep lines, which form as the muscular layer of the face becomes uneven.

Evidence that this must be the case is that the deep wrinkles associated with skin creasing occur only in the areas where muscle is attached to the skin. At the sides of the face there are two sets of chewing muscles that move the jaw. They're not like the other facial muscles- they move the jaw in the same way as the other skeletal muscles move the arms, fingers, etc, they aren't attached to the skin, and there's no wrinkling at the sites of these muscles - they're in the temple and back of the jaw.

There's no line on the skin where the jaw meets the neck, either, even though the skin is permanently bent at a right-angle, and we've been told all our lives that the neck needs a special cream as the skin here is extra delicate. Skin here is free of the muscle and when the muscle contracts or relaxes the adjustment in the skin is distributed evenly over a large area of skin rather than tethered at the site of the muscle itself.

The muscular layer becomes misshapen because the facial muscles are different from the muscles in the rest of the body, far more different than the facial skin is from the rest of the skin. The facial muscles just 'sink' back to their starting position, they have no antagonistic muscles to pull them flat (as a tricep is pulled when the bicep flexes, and vice versa), and they return to their resting shape in a similar way to how a piece of foam springs back after you've pressed your palm into it (turgor, the tendency to resist distortion).

Older people's muscles don't spring back to the face so well. If you bounce your palm up and down on the foam for long enough, eventually it will leave an indentation. In a similar way, areas of furrows and bumps appear on the face where the muscle hasn't fully returned to its shape at rest.

So a face gets permanently wrinkled as you age simply because your muscles are retaining the shape of many expressions all the time. It's not simply that the skin is moulded to the less regular surface of the older muscle…it puckers so it can accommodate the dips and ridges that pull it sharply in one direction or another

This is why Botox works so superbly and injecting collagen or other fillers gives less satisfactory results in deep wrinkles. Filling deep lines in the skin isn't much use because the muscular structure that the skin is fused to is still pulling it awry. The thickness and elasticity of the skin affects the depth of the wrinkle, but this is like saying a thick, elastic tablecloth can be pulled out of shape further before it wrinkles. The skin can disguise the irregularity underneath, but by far the most effective way of smoothing it out is to smooth out the muscles and encourage them to lie flat as they do in youth.

Botox eradicates lines instantly because the muscle flattens when it is relaxed, not really because the muscle is immobilised and prevented from creasing the skin. Once the muscle relaxes fully, deep lines are immediately reduced to traces, not gradually eradicated over the weeks and months like creases dropping from a crumpled dress that you've finally hung up.

People expect facial training to be as different to Botox as it is possible to be. The reasoning is that since paralysing a muscle smooths out wrinkles, making it stronger will increase them. But strengthening the muscles enables them to snap back into shape when they rest. So facial training works in a similar way to Botox because it also works at flattening the underlying muscle so that it more fully regains its resting shape. Facial training is the logical way to approach facial ageing , even if wrinkling was the only thing that counted in this.

However diligent you are and no matter how much money you spend on your face, the deep lines will never lift while the muscular distortion remains. The skin can't lie on the face any other way unless a surgeon pulls out the wrinkles in a face lift.

As it's so obviously the answer to everyone's prayers it seems crazy that everyone isn't working their face like mad, but there are reasons why facial training receives such a mixed press....here are some of them.

People think the exercise gives them wrinkles. When you exercise a muscle by using it to make an expression, it will take a little time, an hour or so, for it to relax and lie completely flat, just as it would if you'd been squinting or puzzling a lot. The difference is that the intensity of the exercise is toning the underlying muscle and encouraging it to behave more like it did when you were younger, while just pulling a face isn't doing anything very much (rather like putting on a hat doesn't develop biceps, or even flexing your biceps doesn't do much for your biceps). The lines etched into the face return to normal in a little while, and the muscles learn to snap back into shape a little better next time With normal smiling or staring, they haven't been trained to do anything.

This has been a problem with facial exercise in the past, though.... It hasn't been demanding enough and progress is slow while the post-exercise lines are a bit alarming and persistent due to the volume of exercise necessary to make any difference to the muscle.

Even now that more effective exercises have been devised using resistance (see below), so that changes in the face are achieved more quickly, people often train too much because they're keen to see changes even faster, so that the muscles hardly get a chance to return to their resting state before they're being worked again, so the temporary lines and bumps which come after you've made the expression seem to be permanent, and people see that the more they do their exercises the worse the problem gets, so naturally they assume that the exercises are giving them wrinkles. They aren't... the muscle underneath is responding to the exercise, but changes in the muscle don't take place while you're training, they happen in the times you rest and recover. People don't have enough of these, until they lose faith and give up their facial training for a day or two, and then the lines disappear entirely and it becomes clear that the face has benefited from the exercise. They then conclude that they look far, far better for not training. But of course, they look good because they did the training in the first place, not because they stopped doing it!

It's also the case that in order to rebuild the skin and muscle tissue more strongly the body will first break down the old muscle and skin fibres. I'm very much indebted to Dave Metzer for pointing out to me that the face will look more or less tired during periods of rebuilding, and again, the heavier the workload the less space there is for the body to recover and look good. Again, people train their hearts out and again, when they stop and the face recovers they think they look so much better for not training their faces.

The method of training in this book is designed to make progress as steady and heartening as possible, so people are actually looking better before they look a lot better. It does this in two ways.

First, the programme succeeds in conditioning the muscles far more thoroughly than in the 'smile very hard' type of facial exercise because you apply really effective resistance to make the muscle work more productively... it's the same principle as weight training This course provides very effective resistance, so that each rumpling of the tissues comes with a big gain in terms of muscle condition, so that improvements are rapid and less time screwing up the face means temporary wrinkles aren't the problem they might be if you were to just use exaggerated expressions.

Secondly, the amount of daily training is very modest... five minutes or less, and you're asked to exercise one part of the face one day, the others the next. This gives your face plenty of time to recover and rebuild, so you stay looking nice. But try always to bear in mind that the effects of an exercise won't show until a few days after you've done it.

Elinor Glyn

This is the novelist Elinor Glyn, who wrote about her own facial exercises and robust treatment of the skin (including scrubbing it with a brush) in 'The Wrinkle Book or, How to Stay Looking Young' (1927). It's not known when the photo on this page was taken, but the picture opposite on page 19 was taken in 1943, she's 78.

Glyn shows how the face responds to intense training and the skin thrives on being tugged and handled. She also shows how well you can do without cutting-edge night cream... her skin is beautiful because she kept it out of the sun. It's not quite accurate to say that nothing on sale will make a really significant difference to your skin's condition... Heavy-duty sunblock with an Ultra (*****) UVA rating are a gift from God. Boots Soltan and La Roche Posay's Anthelios are two examples.

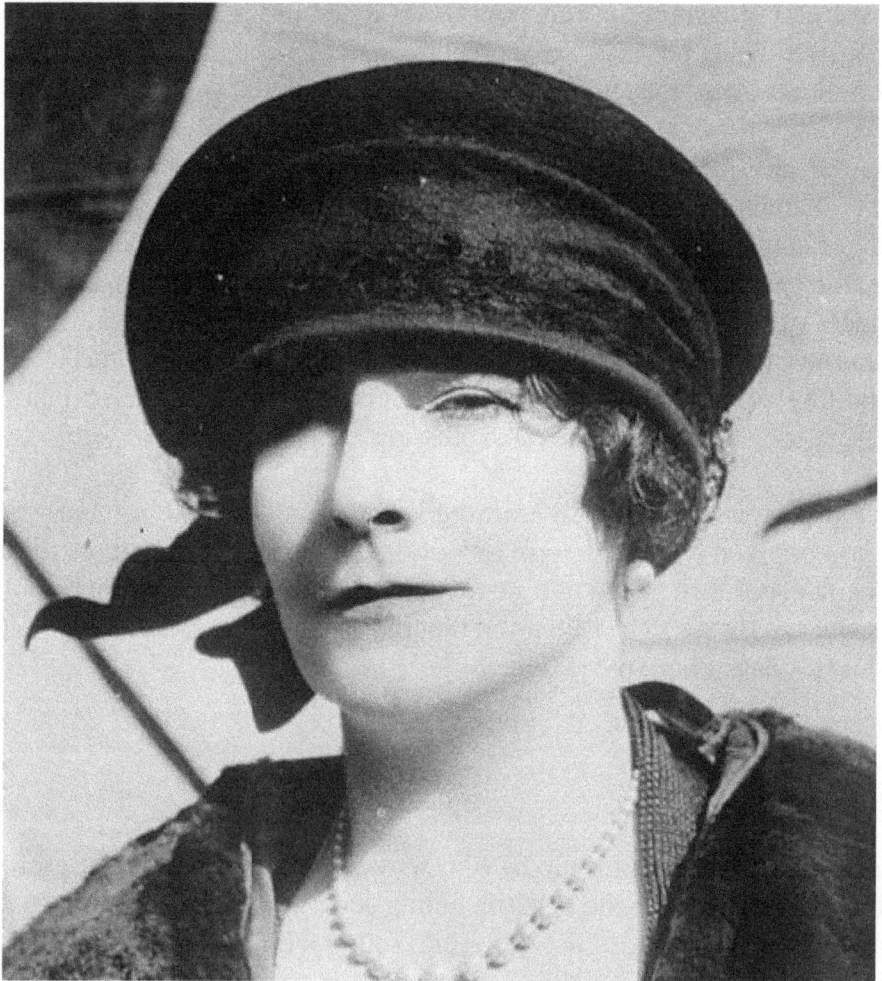

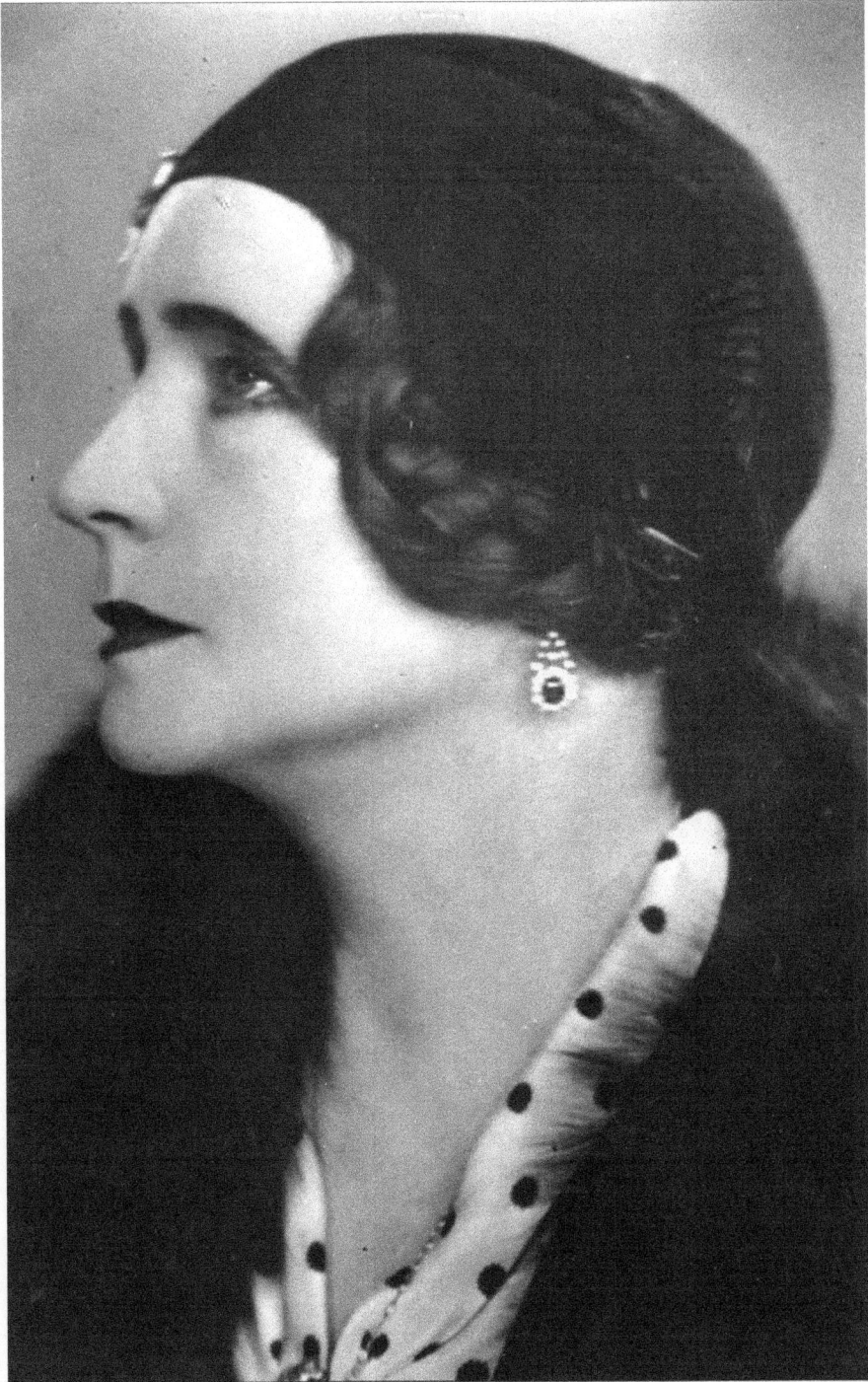

Women deserve to have more than twelve years between
the ages of twenty-eight and forty.

~James Thurber, *Time*, 15 August 1960

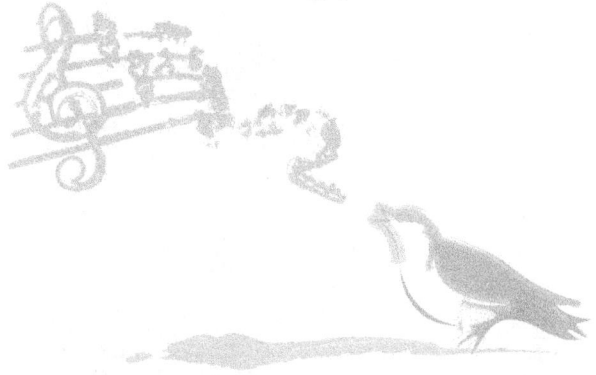

Chapter two
How a face changes

The ageing process follows the same pattern in most cases, and to illustrate that here are two faces so as to compare young and old. The wrinkling described in chapter 1 goes alongside a general movement towards the lower and central areas of the face as the muscles lengthen with lack of exercise and the facial flesh slides down with them.

The shape of a woman's face comes to look more masculine as there's more bulk in the lower areas of a face, and the upper cheeks lose their roundness, partly because fat is lost, but mainly because the cheeks are now low on the face, making big folds from nose to mouth and a heavy jaw line. Bette Davis is the female example in this chapter and her face doesn't look masculine, but it's important to be respectful when talking about this, so the two people being used as examples aged rather well.

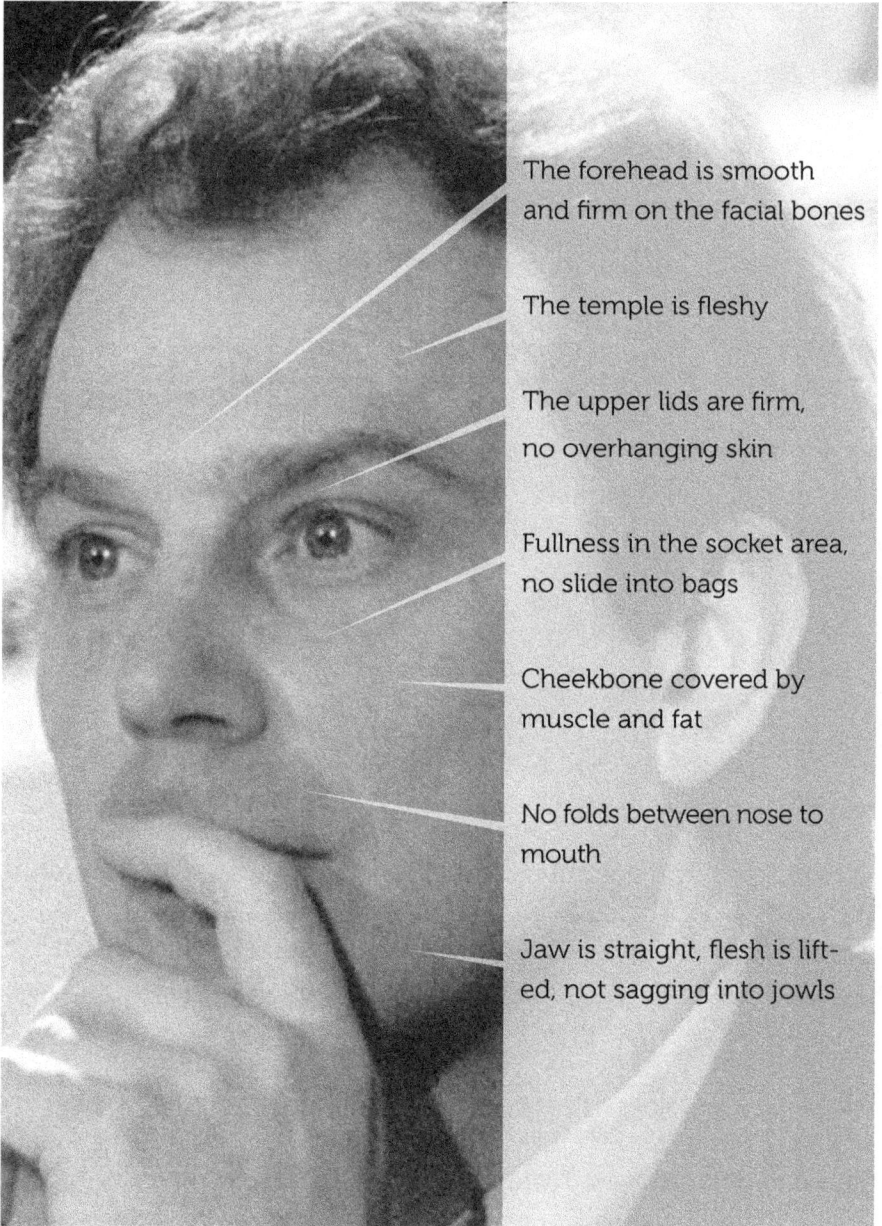

The forehead is smooth and firm on the facial bones

The temple is fleshy

The upper lids are firm, no overhanging skin

Fullness in the socket area, no slide into bags

Cheekbone covered by muscle and fat

No folds between nose to mouth

Jaw is straight, flesh is lifted, not sagging into jowls

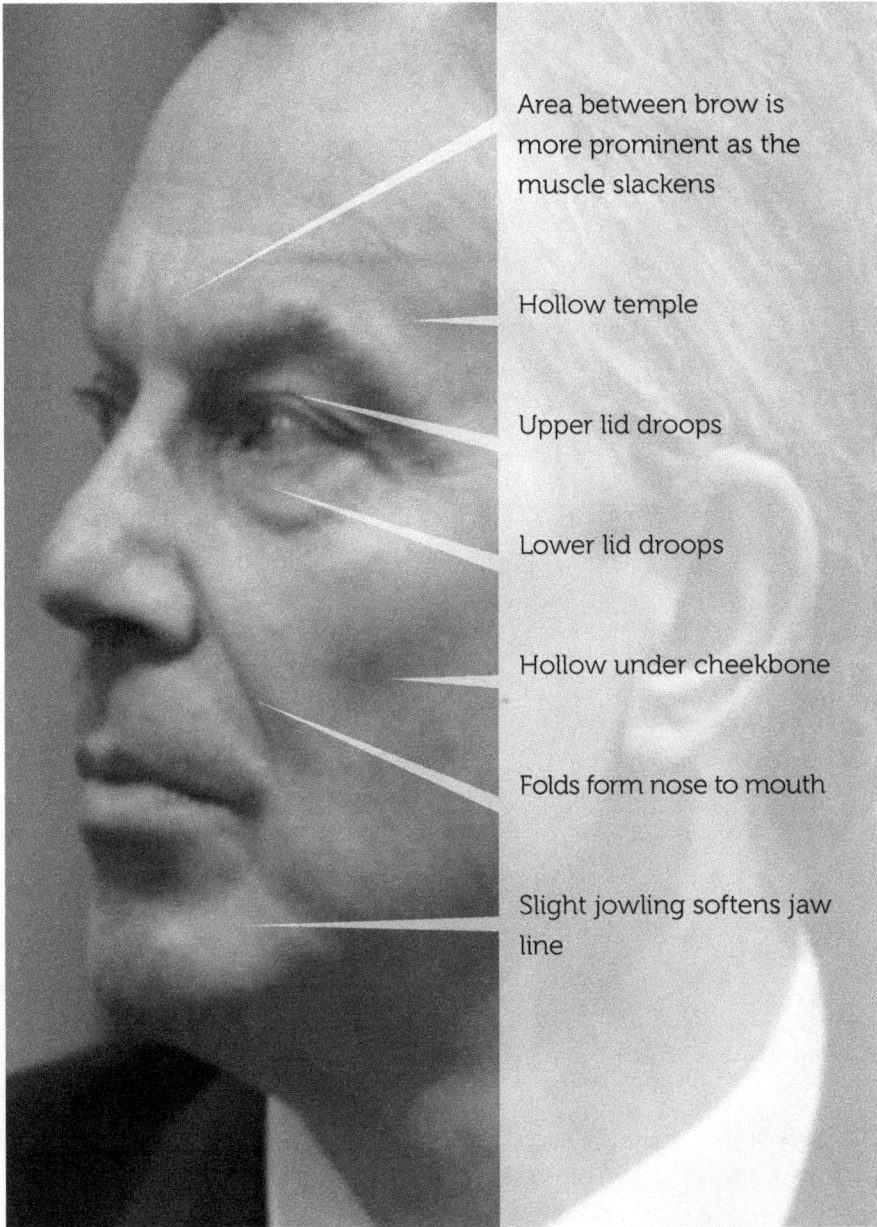

Area between brow is more prominent as the muscle slackens

Hollow temple

Upper lid droops

Lower lid droops

Hollow under cheekbone

Folds form nose to mouth

Slight jowling softens jaw line

Men have an easier time ageing. They have thicker skin and more muscle mass. Tony Blair looks more statesmanlike in later life.

21

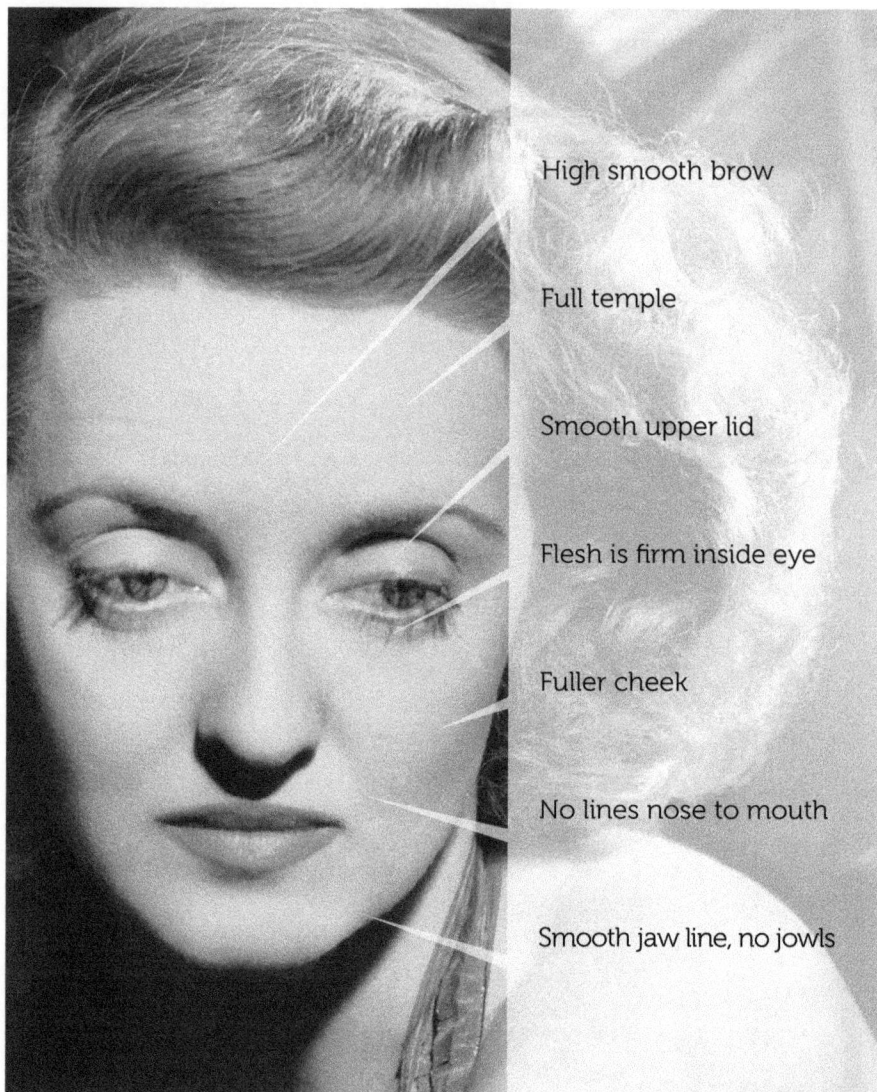

High smooth brow

Full temple

Smooth upper lid

Flesh is firm inside eye

Fuller cheek

No lines nose to mouth

Smooth jaw line, no jowls

Bette Davis looks so cool even a sagging face looks good on her. Below the picture opposite is a rough comparison between the proportions of her younger and older face, younger measurements on the left, older on the right. You see how the forehead is lower (although this isn't obvious in many people because the hairline recedes a little), and the lip-to-chin area is longer as you get older. See also the cover pictures of me for how reversible this change is.

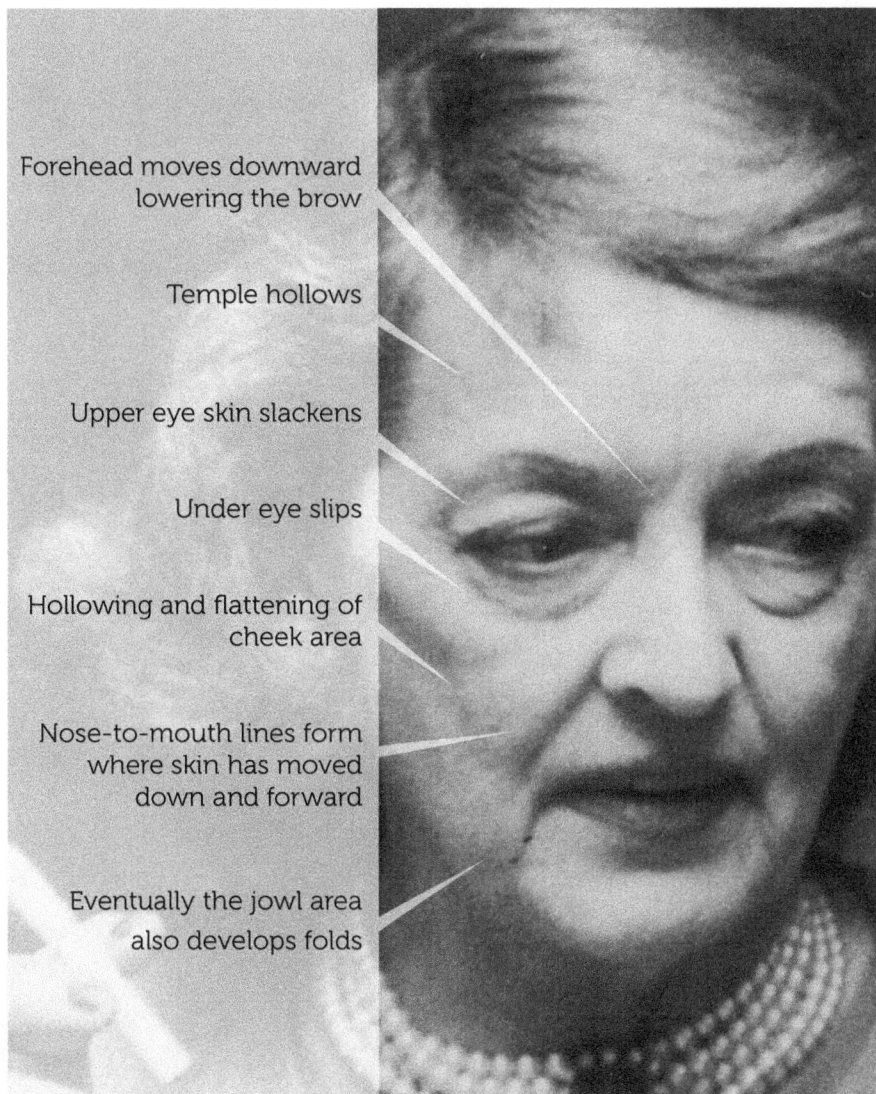

Forehead moves downward
lowering the brow

Temple hollows

Upper eye skin slackens

Under eye slips

Hollowing and flattening of
cheek area

Nose-to-mouth lines form
where skin has moved
down and forward

Eventually the jowl area
also develops folds

Forehead (hairline to
bridge of nose)

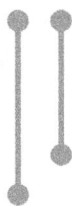

Nose (bridge to tip)

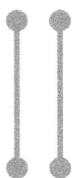

Lower lip to tip of chin

23

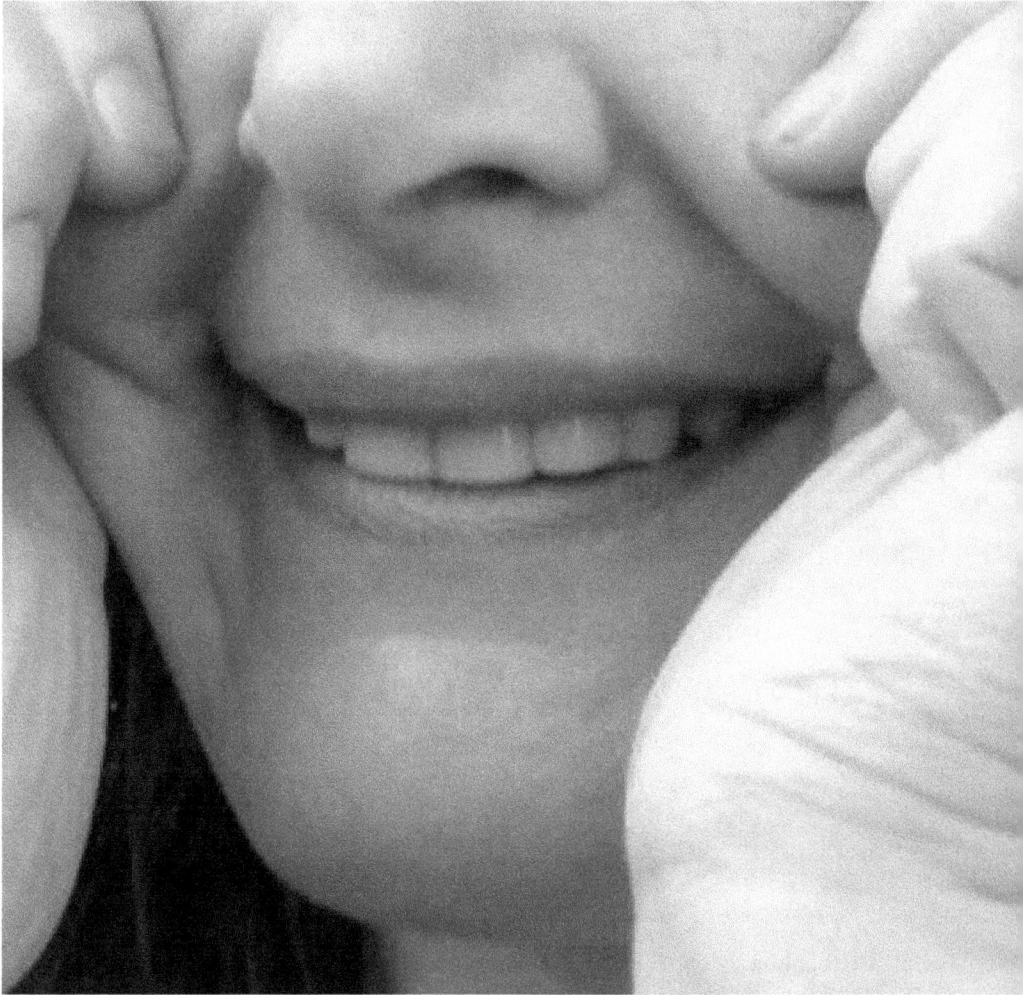

Chapter three
Why the cheeks lift everything

The cheek muscles near the surface of the skin lift and shape the upper cheeks. The diagrams that follow show their position and indicate the direction in which they pull.

As gravity draws the face down and in, jowls and folds from nose-tomouth are formed, and the jaw loses its clean line. You can see from the diagrams that the four superficial cheek muscles radiate like the spokes of a wheel over a 90-degree angle.

Much of what you think of as the cheekbone is muscular tissue, and training these four muscles will rebuild the contours of this area as well as lifting the face up and out along different gradients.

The deeper muscles (just two of these) are represented on the facial bones on the left hand side of the diagram. The caninus, from its position deeper beneath the surface, also lifts up the face.The buccinator, amongst its other virtues, will pull the sagging areas of skin horizontally from the middle of the face when it is toned and firm.

So there is a second layer of muscles pulling outwards towards the perimeter of the face, crossing under the first, and supporting it. In any face, improving the condition of the cheek muscles can to some extent reverse the changes described.

If you just look at the diagrams overleaf, you'll see immediately how this must be. All the muscles that determine the shape of the cheeks are to some degree lip elevators, and pull the tissue from the central areas of the face up and out towards the fixed bony points of attachment.

Superficial muscles

1)   Levator labii (vertical) [1]
2)   Zygomaticus minor (diagonal, small) [2]
3)   Zygomaticus major (diagonal, large)
4)   Risorius (horizontal)

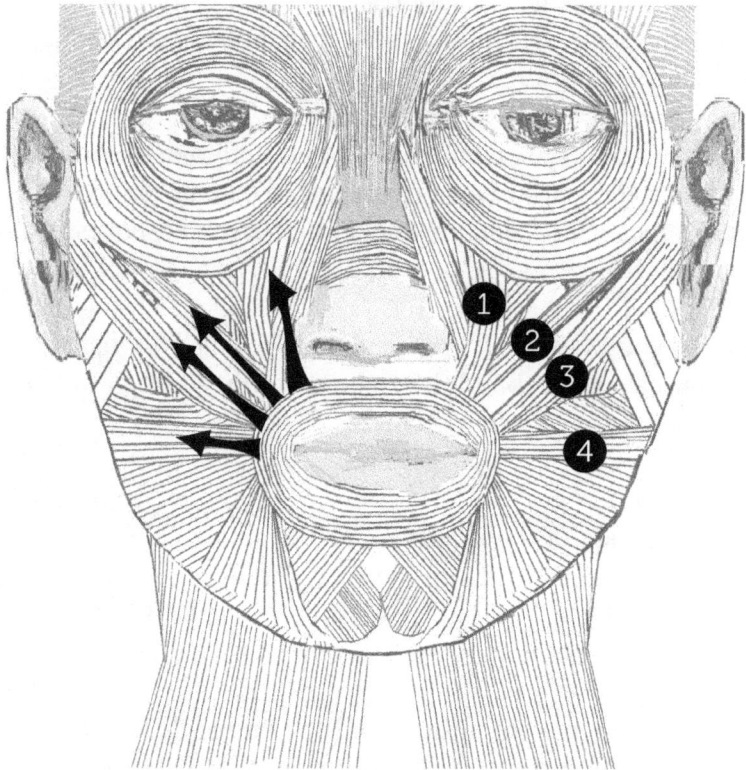

[1]. The levator labii properly refers to a multi-headed muscle, but here the term is applied to just one of its heads, i.e. the caput infra-orbital. This is to simplify, and is inaccurate!

[2]. This is sometimes considered a separate muscle, or another head of the levator labii (the caput zygomaticum). It's a separate muscle here, again, because it's slightly easier to consider it in this way.

The superficial muscles
from the side.

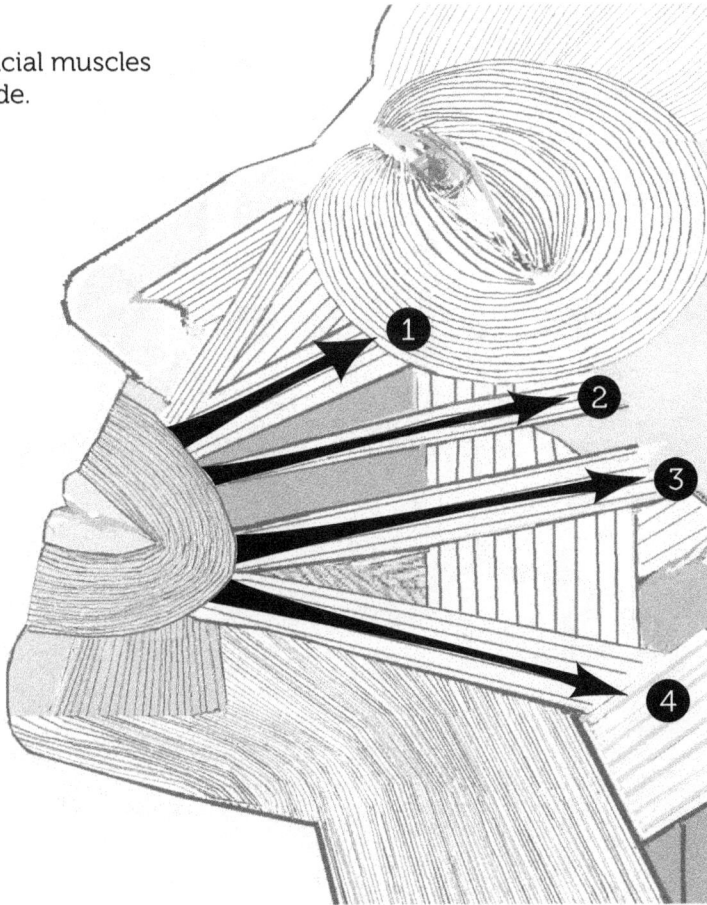

Deep Muscles

Deep muscles shown on the skull, although only one end is fixed to the skull…
all the cheek muscles become merged with the lip muscles rather than having
a distinct end-point.

5)   Caninus (deep muscle)
6)   Buccinator (broad cheek muscle)

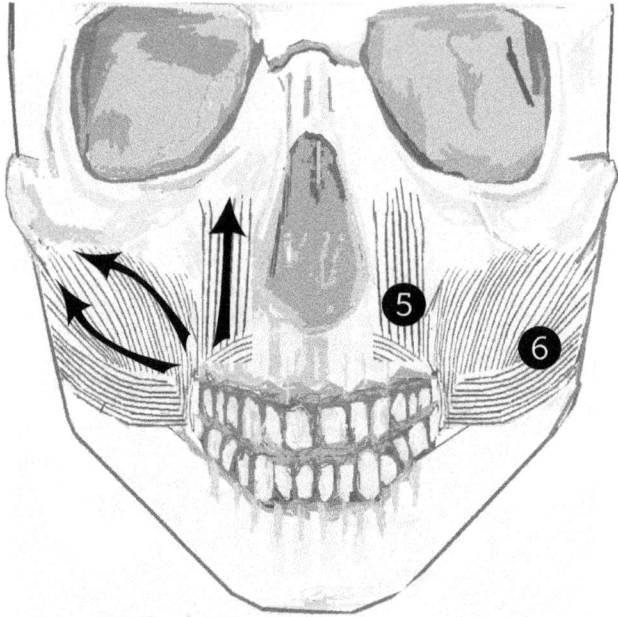

The deeper facial muscles
from the side.

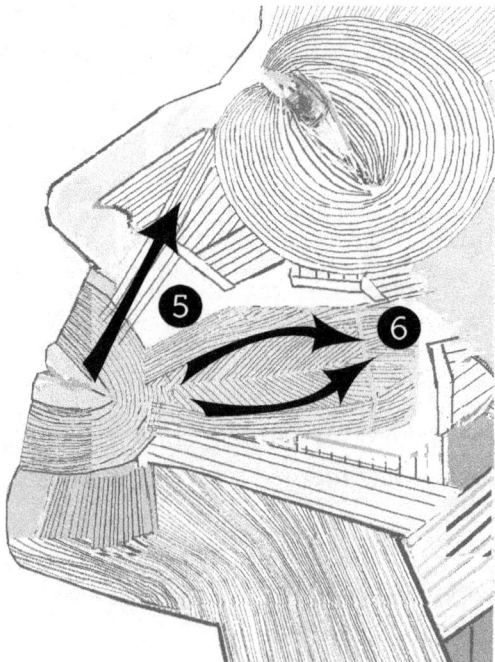

1. Levetor Labiii

The muscle Levator Labii is a vertical muscle that draws the central area of the lip up towards the mid area of the eye socket and rebuilds the shape of the front of the cheek. It's a thick chunk of muscle and contributes to restoring the volume lost as fat stores diminish. The upper lip is lifted in the middle, showing the teeth more when you smile or talk. Thin lips usually happen because the lip/cheek muscles cease to hold them up and they roll into the mouth. Yikes.

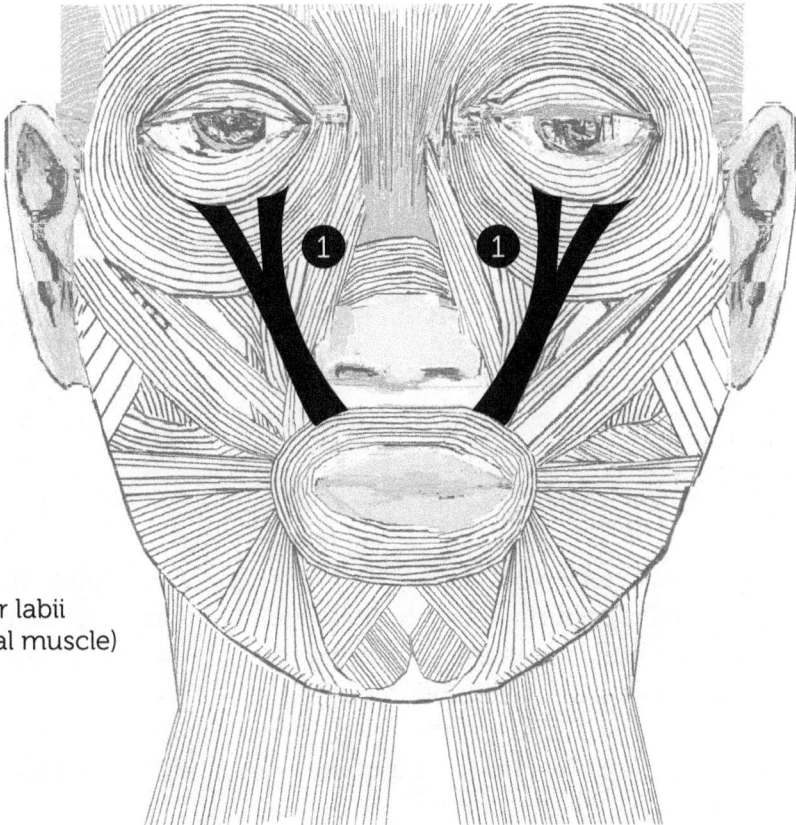

Levator labii
(vertical muscle)

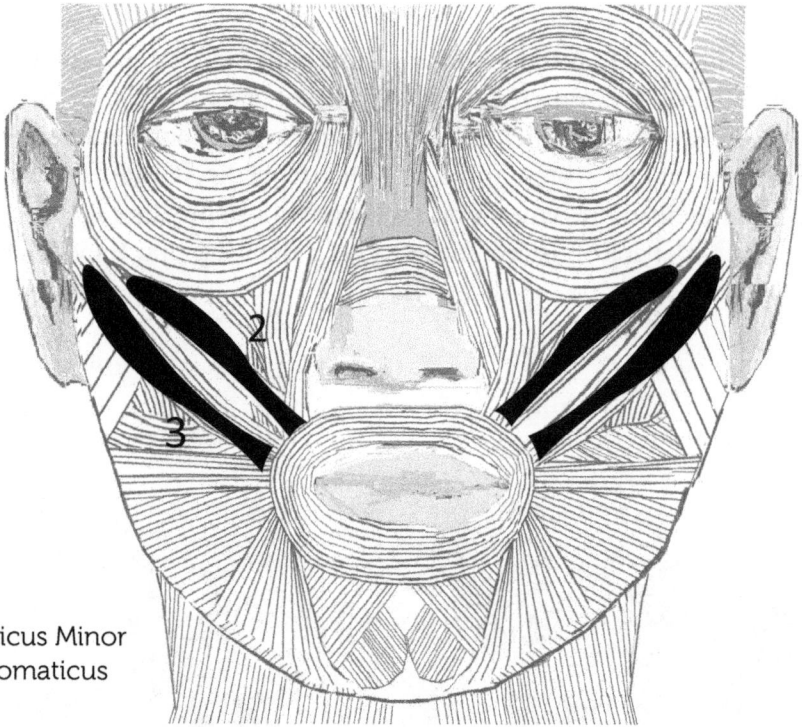

Zygomaticus Minor
(2) & Zygomaticus
Major (3)

It has its origin under the eye socket, a proportion of its fibres attach to the upper jaw and some attach to the cheekbone. Hence it looks Y shaped. Its fibres merge with those circling the mouth (orb. oris) .

2. Zygomaticus Minor

The Zygomaticus Minor is the smaller diagonal muscle, that pulls the outer lip towards the temple, and builds the cheek area high on the cheekbone. It originates on the cheekbone. Again, it terminates, or rather fizzles out, at the mouth muscle, where the two muscles lose their identity.

Its position between the two bigger muscles means a little extra mass added to it fills out the entire cheekbone area. The upper lip is lifted at the corners, crinkling the eyes. Using the inner face includes companions in a smile, at its most emphatic the nose is wrinkled.

The Zygomaticus major-only smile is used all the time in advertising. It avoids wrinkling or narrowing of the eyes as happens when the other smiling muscles are used, but I think that more than this the zygomaticus major-only smile is happy, but not friendly. You're invited to admire this kind of smile, not return it, because it's aimed at your aspirations, presenting you with a world you're not part of. It's someone smiling down indulgently at you, not an exchange between equals. Raising muscles 1 and 2 is a gesture on top of the happy smile, to show that you're smiling at or with or for someone.

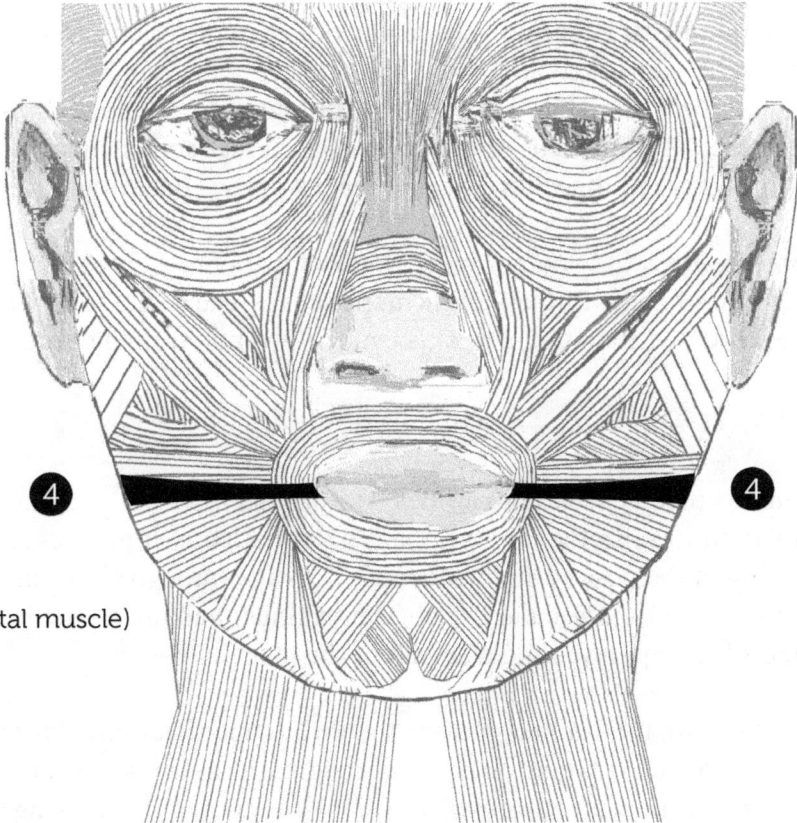

Risorius
(horizontal muscle)

3. Zygomaticus Major

The Zygomaticus Major is the larger diagonal muscle that draws the lip wide to the side. It arises at the outer area of the cheekbone, and ends mixed with the mouth muscles.

When it's exercised, tissue is grasped horizontally, and the muscle moves the corner of the mouth in a shallow diagonal towards the ear. That is, using it produces a broad, happy smile, and building it restores the contour of the upper, outer cheek.

4. Risorius

The Risorius is more or less horizontal, moves the corner of the lip towards the ear lobe and it retracts the lips, making what is often described as a ghastly grin. It maintains a tension between its origin in the thick, strong chewing muscles at the rear of the jaw, and where it ends in the mouth area. The first three muscles discussed in this chapter all build outwards to give volume to the upper face. Zygomaticus minor and major can retract the lips, this muscle instead draws the midface inwards to create a groove under the cheekbone.

This line creates what you normally think of as defined cheekbones. The risorius emphasises the fullness of the upper cheek and at the same time gives the face structure. It distinguishes a beautiful woman from a beautiful child.

5. Caninus

The Caninus (deep cheek muscle) lies beneath the layer of the radiating muscles. It's used to raise the upper lip and bare the teeth. It also redresses the lengthening of the nose-to-lip that occurs with age through the usual process of gravity acting on muscular areas. The caninus maintains tone in the central areas of the lip, revealing as much of the teeth as possible.

In the long term, the caninus presses the three superficial muscles outwards as training makes it bigger and stronger, greatly diminishing nose-mouth lines. with a little work it's possible to make a considerable change in this

32

muscle both in its size (filling out the area beneath the nose-to-mouth fur-row), and in its tone (nicely held upper lip).

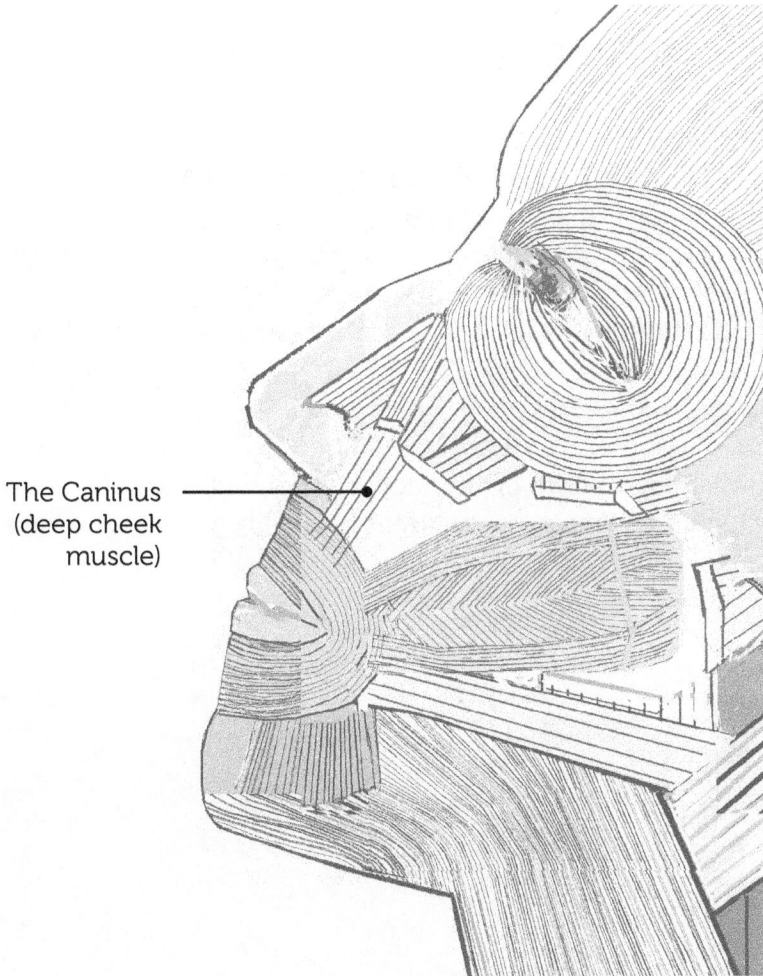

The Caninus
(deep cheek
muscle)

---

[3]. French is spoken from the front of mouth, and the upper lip is raised frequently in form-ing its words. The on-off caninus signal is very attractive to people of the opposite sex. Germanic languages make more sounds with the back of the mouth and throat, the lip remaining relatively immobile.

Expression-wise, the snarl produced by contracting the caninus is without an obvious charm. But its signals powerful messages. It expresses passion and desire as well as menace, hence the fascination of brooding men, and Elvis, and Frenchwomen[3]. You might not always want to be light-hearted and smiling, although we are aiming to feel contented and easy with ourselves, it's good to retain your bite.

6. Buccinator

The Buccinator, or broad muscle is the other muscle of the cheek that lies close to the bone, although this is a bit misleading as it has areas where it's the only layer of muscle, so also close to the surface. In fact the fleshy area of the cheek is mainly comprised of this muscle plus a layer of skin, so maintaining firmness and thickness is invaluable for keeping a strong structure to the face.

It's a large muscle, and it pulls the fleshy area of the cheek inward (ie toward the skull, not toward the middle of the face). Its original purpose was to keep food in the mouth and it can be used for blowing, hence its Latin name, meaning 'trumpet- blower'.

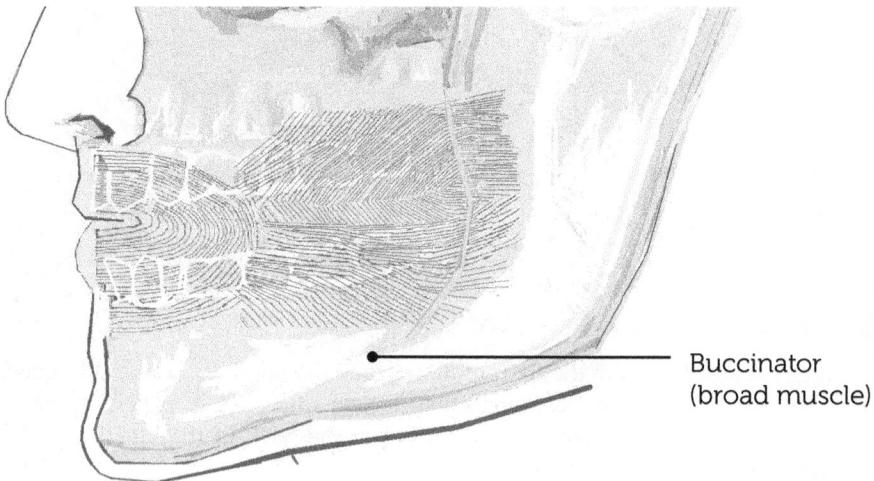

Buccinator
(broad muscle)

It connects the upper jawbone with the lower, attaching to the layer of tendon near the back of the mouth. As well as covering the mid-cheek area, its fibres also extend into the large circular muscle around the mouth (orbicularis oris), where they pass across the upper and lower lip, merging with the other muscles that converge here.

Often the face takes on a sculpted look quite early in your training. Some people, especially younger people or those who think of themselves as having chubby faces, like the look of the cheek when it's pulled in beneath the cheekbones, and have achieved the look they hoped for. If this happens, stop building the buccinator and train it only occasionally so as to maintain the tone of the muscle.

For some people the effect of sculpting is more than they would like, and they can stop training for the buccinators altogether for a while so they relax a little. You don't need to train every muscle of your face to the max.

The Buccinator is not expressive as such, but the fact that the risorius and zygomaticus major muscles touch upon it or cross it gives it the glorious quality of raising a smile out of nowhere.

When you've been training for a little while, try this. Touch your front teeth with the corners of your lips, very gently. Now use your buccinators to try to touch your teeth a little further back with the inside of your cheek. The lips don't have to remain in contact with the front teeth. Now gently try to touch the teeth with the cheek further and further back until the very back of your cheek is pressing against the very back of the teeth. It doesn't matter if you can't actually make contact, just trying is fine.

Now try to press back further still with the cheek muscles and feel the smile welling up inside you as the buccinator lifts up the zygomaticus muscle. Maybe you feel like laughing, too. That's the risorius. It has the capacity to trigger laughter as well as express it.

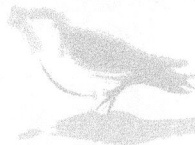

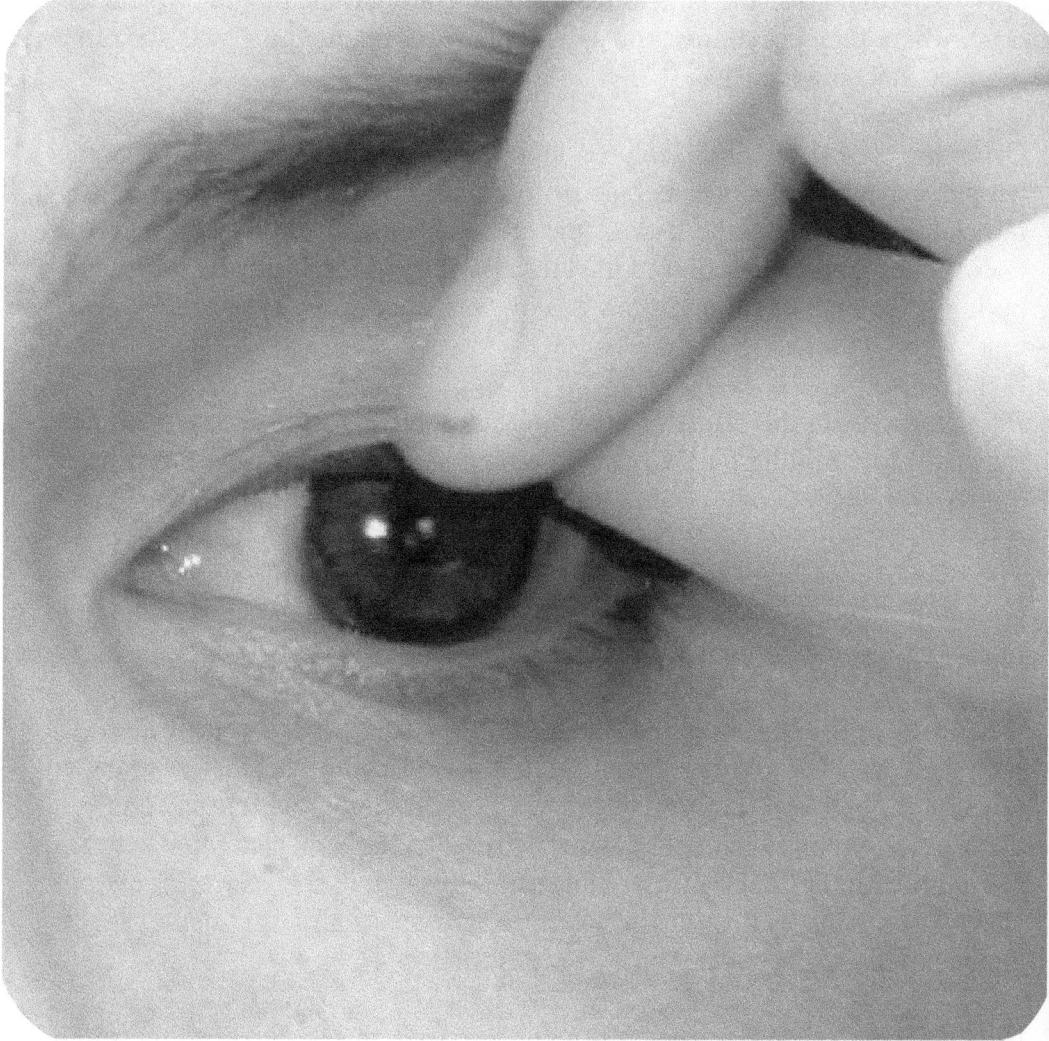

Chapter four

The muscles that lift everything else

For a long time I exercised only one muscle in order to firm and sharpen the jawline.

7. Platysma

The Platysma (flat throat muscle) covers a huge surface area from the upper chest, up either side of the neck and over the jaw to the lower areas of the face. It's a thin muscle, but it has a positive effect

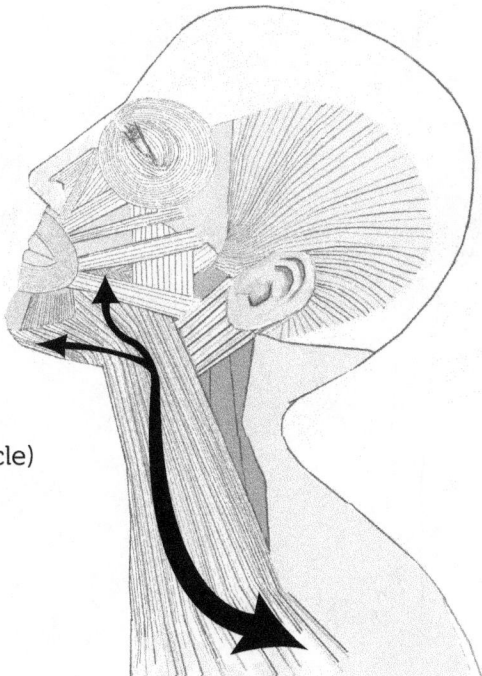

Platysma
(flat throat muscle)

37

on the appearance of every area it covers. In the upper chest, the platysma flows from the pectoral fascia (the thick membrane that covers the large chest muscles). Firming and slightly thickening the platysma gives a nice fullness to the upper chest. which often looks bony as fat levels drop.

On the throat, the platysma covers the muscles that criss-cross over the neck, and the thicker fibres prevent them from showing through.

The diagram shows the mass of cord-like muscles that lie beneath the platysma. They're very prominent when the flat throat muscle is weakened and thin. Plus the front edges of the flat throat muscles curl outwards creating a pair of vertical ridges that look like tendons. The tauter the muscle, the less

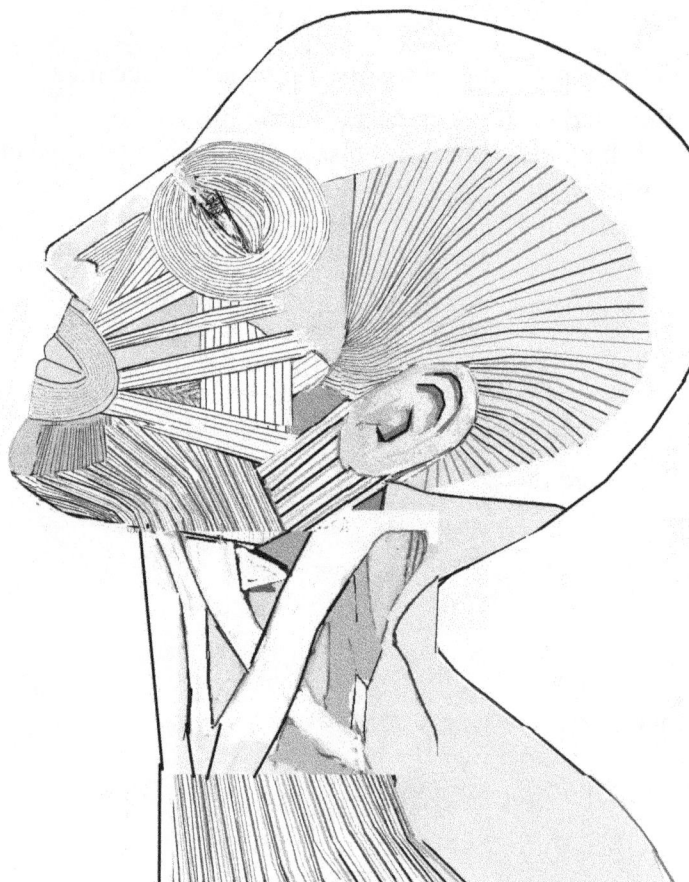

scope there is for it to curl. Where the platysma extends over the jaw on to the lower part of the face, the muscle fibres are inserted into the skin at many points all over the surface, so that when conditioned it will lie flat against the jaw, pulling the skin with it, and preventing the facial tissue that's been dragged down the face by gravity from collecting there.

Although maintaining the platysma in good condition is really important, it's worth remembering that one of its functions is to turn the mouth downward. It's much better to contract it by retracting the jaw, so you don't engage the other mouth downturner, the triangularis.

Once you get used to the feeling of gently retracting the jaw (the temporalis is involved also) and maintaining the angle between your jawbone and neck you'll notice how it affects how you feel. While the cheek muscles are cheerful and friendly, the jaw allows you to feel controlled and dignified, assured when you lack confidence and graceful where you feel unsure in your surroundings. Vive la platysma.

8. Orbicularis oculis

The orbicularis oculi is the large circular muscle around the eye. The large eye muscle can be divided into two parts that can be moved independently.

The orbital (socket) part of the muscle is made up of concentric rings which shrink as the fibres shorten, narrowing the eye in the process.

If you imagine each ring of fibre becoming thicker, there will be an increase in size in the temple area, over the cheekbone and under the eye in the area known as the tear trough (the channel that carries tears away when they leave the eyes). All these areas, plus the eye socket itself, hollow as you get older, partly from loss of fat and from muscle atrophy, partly because the force exerted by gravity encourages the tissue to slide downwards, causing a hooded area above the eye and a hollow beneath it.

The palpebral (eyelid) portion governs the lids themselves and consists of fibres running in concentric curves above and below the eye. There is not really a muscle that opens the lower lid, so the condition of the under-eye area

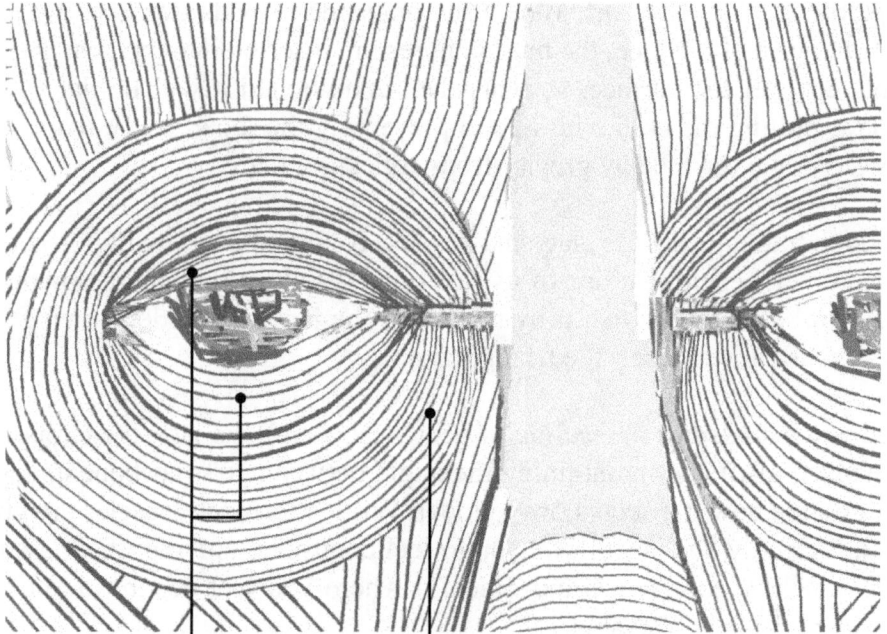

Palpebral
(eyelid) portion

Orbital
(socket) portion

is mainly determined by the condition of the orbicularis oculi that closes it. Wrinkled skin beneath the eyes looks worse because the muscle is drooping and everything has sagged into a bag. There's no muscle tissue to smooth out the skin and fill out the area.

Of all the areas you're training, your eyes are the area that will respond first. The muscles are almost fused to the skin. It's a relatively fast process to firm the muscle, and the skin will automatically flatten with it and the area will look toned and youthful again.

9. Levator labii

The levator labii is the upper lid muscle that opens the eye.

Tightening the skin around the eyes surgically can sometimes make them look smaller, but training this muscle makes them look bigger. I've never

40

levator palpebrae

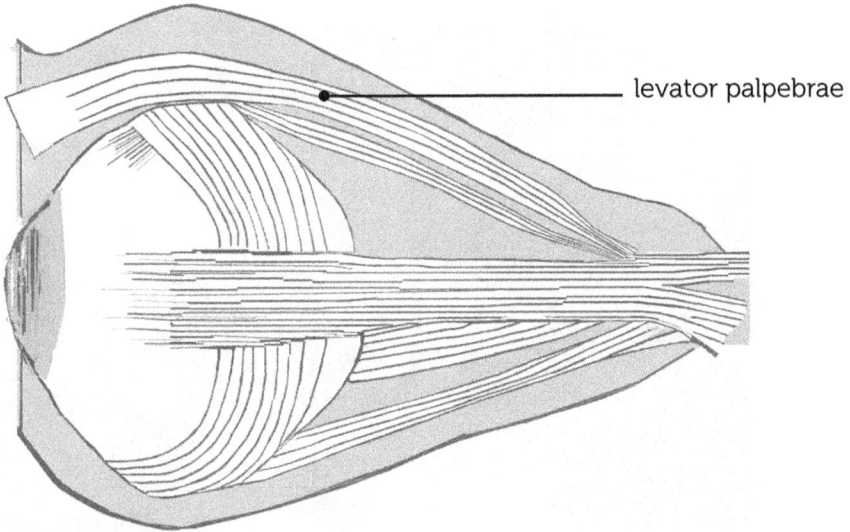

heard of any other method, surgical or otherwise, of doing this. The levator palpebrae can be quite weak initially. It takes two or maybe three sessions, possibly more, before the exercise becomes easy to perform, and people leave it out because it seems too small to make a significant difference to the face. It is not too small! If you can't do it, just pretend you can and do something as close as you can manage. It soon becomes easy to do properly, and I mean three or four sessions.

When you need to feel focused and attentive, you can perform a few repetitions of the exercise for this muscle and notice how wide your eyes feel and how steady your gaze feels and how well you can concentrate.

10. Orbicularis oculis

The orbicularis oris is the large muscle that circles the mouth, and I don't exercise it at all, with the exception of one specific portion of it. It's a mixed blessing because building the area under the lips themselves produces fuller lips and a nice firmness, while training the outer rings and increasing their size will have a few undesirable effects.

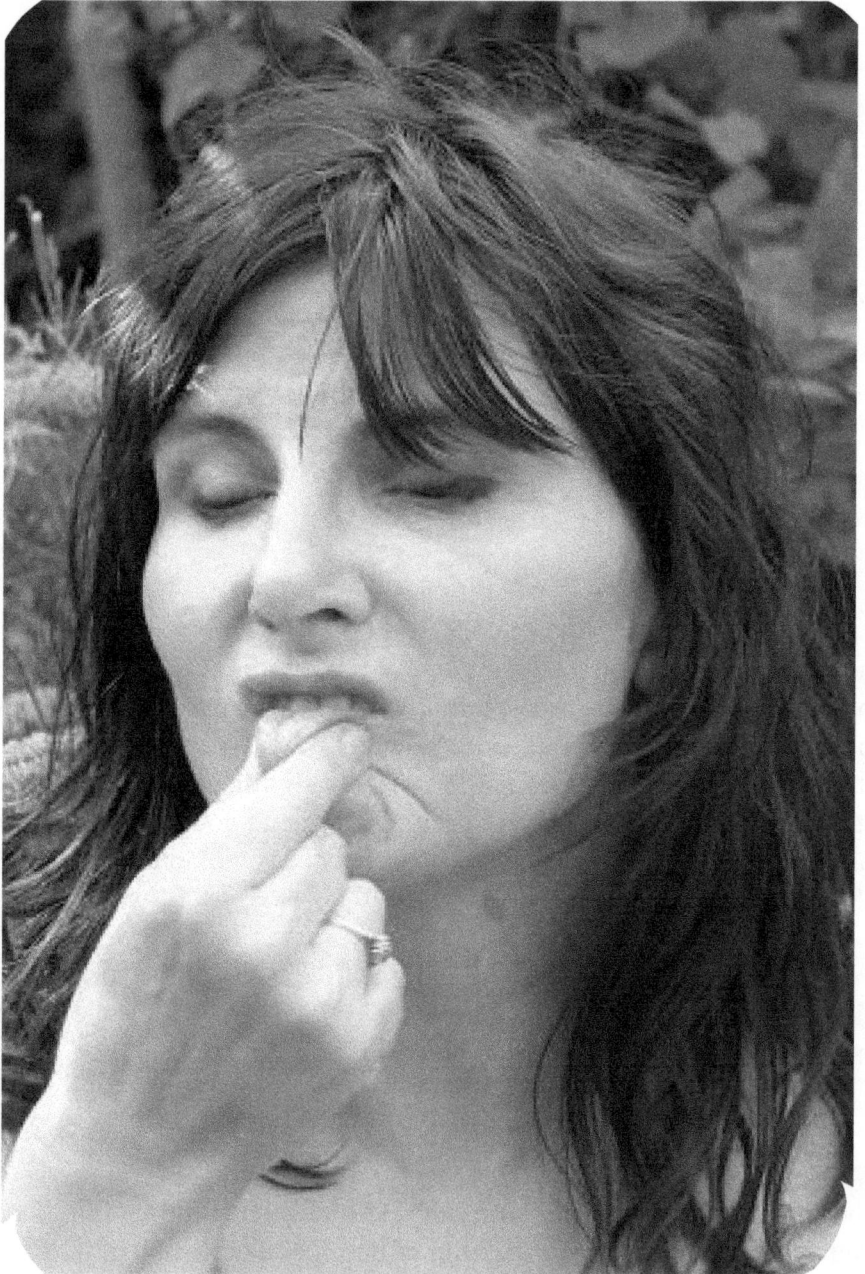

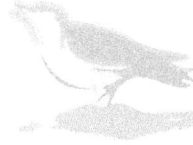

Chapter five
The rest of the face

11. Frontalis

The Frontalis is the flattish, muscle of the forehead, its roughly rectangular shape formed by two distinct halves unified by a central muscular link between the brows. Its function is to raise the eyebrows and move the scalp back. It's attached to a layer beneath the skin so that the skin moves with it, and doesn't attach to any of the facial bones.

Many people, maybe you, immobilise the frontalis with muscle relaxing injections which smooth the forehead, and do so much to rejuvenate the appearance that it's understandable if you want to go on with them. If you want to keep using Botox, that's fine, just don't try to do the forehead exercise (obviously).

Even though the appeal of Botox is clear, there are a couple of reasons to choose facial training instead, the most important being the obvious: facial training will allow total freedom of movement in the brow area. The freedom to move the face is a pleasure, and paralysis in the brow area will make some expressions less easy in every sense. Part of the joy of facial training is the sense of liberty it can give you… you can feel confident in any light or at any distance that your face looks fine, and having irregular movement in the forehead could challenge this confidence.

Galea Aponeurotica
(tendon like layer)

Frontalis

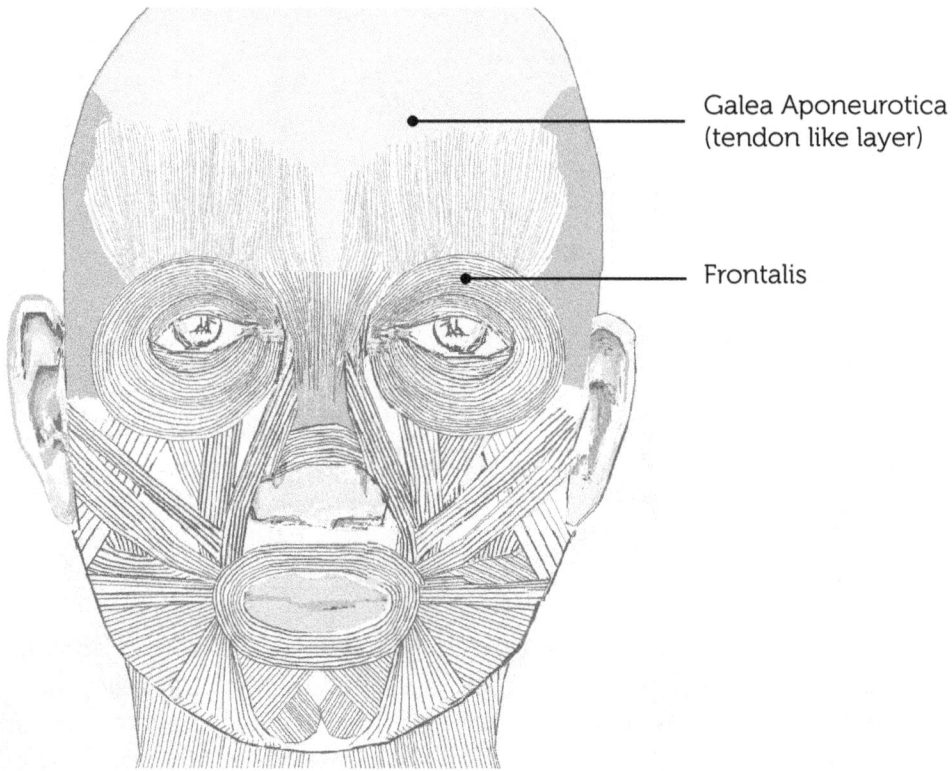

A second reason: after several years of Botox, some people are getting a curiously flat forehead instead of a feminine curved one, and which can make the eyebrows droop a little bit-- it's not too disastrous though.

The diagram shows the large surface area of the broad sheet of tendon that covers the majority of the scalp. The temporalis (shaded) and the muscles of the ears cover the sides of the head, but the scalp is not muscular as such. The sinewy area is moved by the forehead muscles at the front, and a smaller area of muscle at the back of the scalp (the occipitalis). If you Botox the muscles that raise the brows, a large area of your head is immobilised.

Facial trainers often feel very happy about the condition of their hair a few weeks into their schedule. This may be because their facial training is part of a general commitment to their health, or because they just be feel more positive because their face feels nice and they look pretty. But it's also possible that stimulating the scalp with the brow exercises has been beneficial, and that preventing the scalp from moving at all may not be. Having said this, this programme rather sidesteps the forehead (see chapter 7).

But the corrugator (frown) muscles can be immobilised, as they're surprisingly small for a muscle that alters the expression so dramatically, and besides, they're covered by the frontalis muscle, so that any atrophy is covered by an increase in the thickness there. But the strengthening of the other facial muscles and a happier expression makes people less and less likely to use the corrugators unconsciously, and over time they will weaken anyway. It's nice to frown now and then to show people you can, and as you begin to look fabulous it's quite gratifying that people can't put it down to someone else's work. For the record, here is an illustration of the shape and location of the corrugator muscles. Now don't concern yourself with it at all.

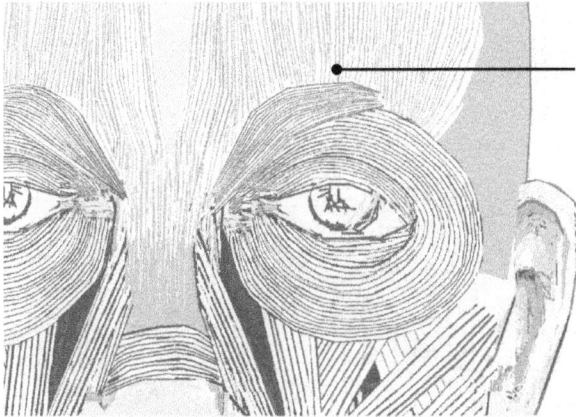

Corrugator muscle
(orbicularis oculis
cut away)

12 & 13. Temporalis

The Temporalis and the masseters are chewing muscles that connect the lower jaw to the upper areas of the skull. They're a special case because they have no attachment to the skin (that is, they're skeletal muscles like those that move the arms, legs and so on). They both raise the jaw, and strengthening them really does allow you to effortlessly hold the jaw close to the upper face, shortening the mid- and lower face instantly. It's one of the facial changes you can't put your finger on, but when it's improved the difference is really striking.

The masseter is a band of muscle running from the upper jaw to the back of the lower jaw, with a deeper layer of muscle making the same attachment slightly closer to the jaw hinge and largely hidden by the superficial portion. The two portions of the masseter are meshed together by the time they reach their area of insertion on the upright part of the jaw. Together they occupy a very large area at the perimeter of the face.

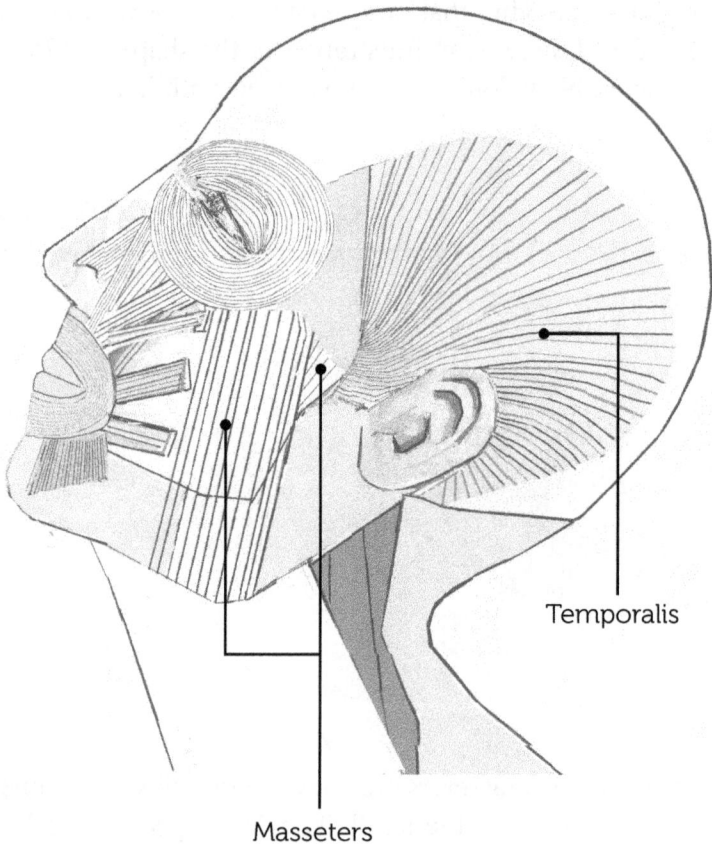

Temporalis

Masseters

The temporalis is the fan-shaped area at the perimeter of the face, which looks as though it is spreading over the temple and extending into the hairline, although technically the muscle fibres go in an inward direction, not radiating from the lower jaw but converging toward it. This area of the muscle is fixed rigidly to the skull and will not move as such, only increase in size. The fibres begin at the furthest points of the fan and converge into a tendon-like structure. They terminate at the front upper corner of the lower jaw.

Building the perimeter of the face counterbalances the inward pull exerted by the trained buccinator and adds width to the face. Given the large size of the chewing muscles, even a little increase in the thickness of either will produce significant muscle mass to compensate for the loss of fat, bone and muscle that's taken place. Building the outer areas of the face will of course cause a slight outward shift of the face.

The jaw hinge is the only area it's possible to damage in the course of facial training. Any muscle that's overworked will recover in a short time without intervention, but the jaw is vulnerable in the same way as the joints of the body, so you may prefer to leave these exercises out. I was cavalier about exercising this area in my early months of training, and still had great things happen to my face. When I began to add occasional exercises for the jaw muscles though, I did notice a marked improvement. Ask your doctor.

Their purpose is to chew, not to communicate or express emotion, but they're used in challenging situations as clenched teeth . It's not desirable to grit the teeth, but the temporalis retracts the jaw as well as raising it. If you feel the need to clench the teeth, try retracting the jaw in a gentle and controlled manner (in conjunction with the platysma...see above).and feel how the determination you're feeling becomes a sense of composure and quiet self confidence. Retracting the jaw seems to draw the head back into line with the body, and the shoulders glide downwards, elongating the neck. The movement brings the entire body into balance and brings to light your feelings of self-worth. It gives you mastery over hurdles and peaceable equality with people.

There are four additional muscles that benefit from occasional attention. They're rather small and only need a little work to keep them firm.

14. Procerus

The Procerus is the area between the brows that pulls the forehead straight down, as opposed to the corrugator that knits the brows together. If overdeveloped it can look quite cro-magnon, which is not good at all on women and not that great on men, either. But it can't be neglected altogether because its fibres are enmeshed with those of the skin. A degree of tone is necessary to avoid the procerus sagging and pulling the skin down with it, creating a slack patch in the middle of your face.

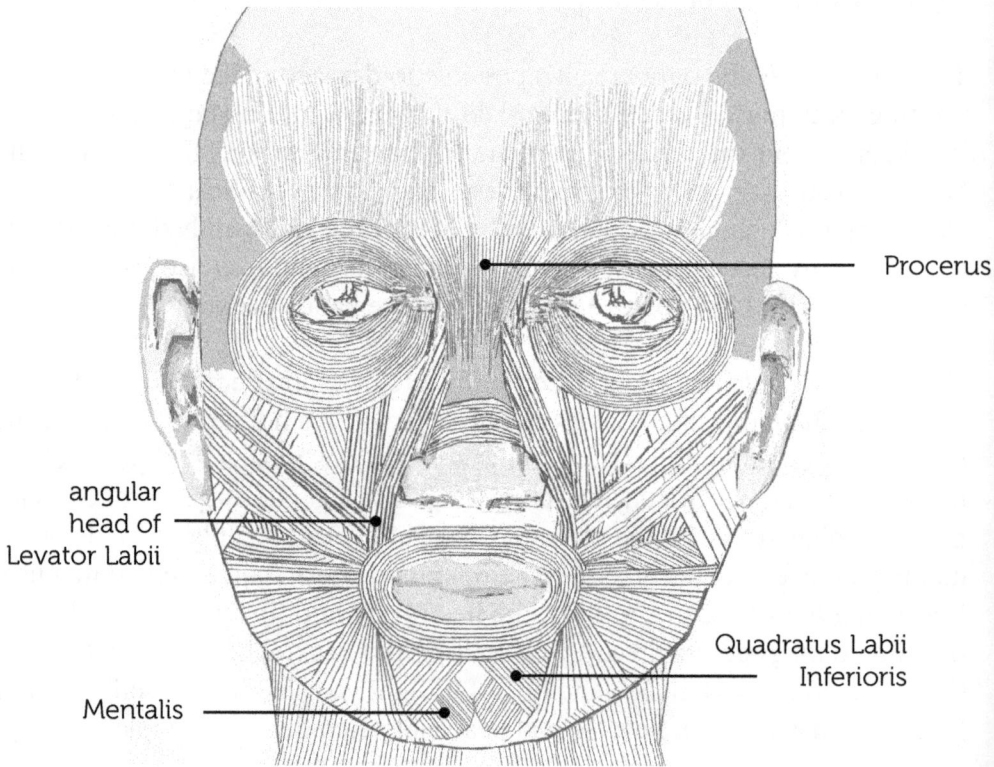

15. Levator Labii (angular head)

A second part of the Levator Labii muscle, the angular head, runs alongside the vertical cheek muscle that is number 1 in the main list. It's called the angular head because it pulls the angle (sloping areas) of the mouth. It has the function of wrinkling the nose, and fills in the area between nose and cheek muscles so that the front of the face is nicely padded. It also assists in pulling up the upper lip, showing teeth etc. . It's located at the side of the nose and joins the vertical muscle to form a decent mass that then inserts into the orbicularis oris (the circular mouth muscle).

16. Quadratus Labii inferioris

The Quadratus Labii inferioris draws the lip corners down. It's much better to have more strength in the lip upturners that are at the top of this list than in the group of less happy muscles to which these belong. The triangularis is another, but that muscle is closely involved with the platysma and will get enough training when the platysma is exercised. The quadratus labii inferioris needs its own exercise every now and then to keep it firm though.

17. Mentalis

The Mentalis is a little muscle that pulls the chin up towards the lower lip and makes dimples it. It doesn't need a lot of training because it's so tiny, but toning it does pull the chin up and reduce the distance between lower lip and the tip of the chin. You don't notice this area has got older until training reverses it.

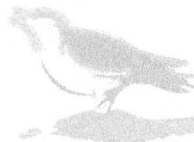

Day one exercises

Every other day if possible, or at least try to do this set of exercises twice a week.

The first two exercises are designed to sculpt the face.

that is, to encourage the flesh to hug the bone .

structure. Most people would welcome a sharper

jawline, but a very sculpted cheek might not be so desirable.

The later exercises are for spot-training, for improving the look

and feel of small local areas of the face.

Exercise 1
Lift cheeks 1

Type. A structural exercise, i.e. an exercise to revive the muscular structures that support the face. Lifts midface vertically.

Muscle. Levator labii.

Result. Lifts mid-face vertically.

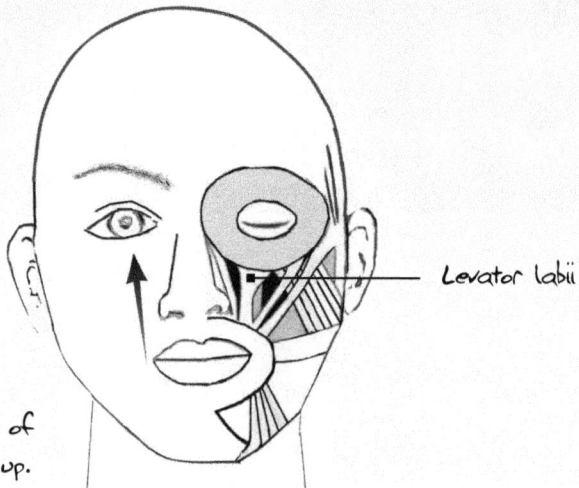

Levator labii

Lifts corners of mouth straight up.

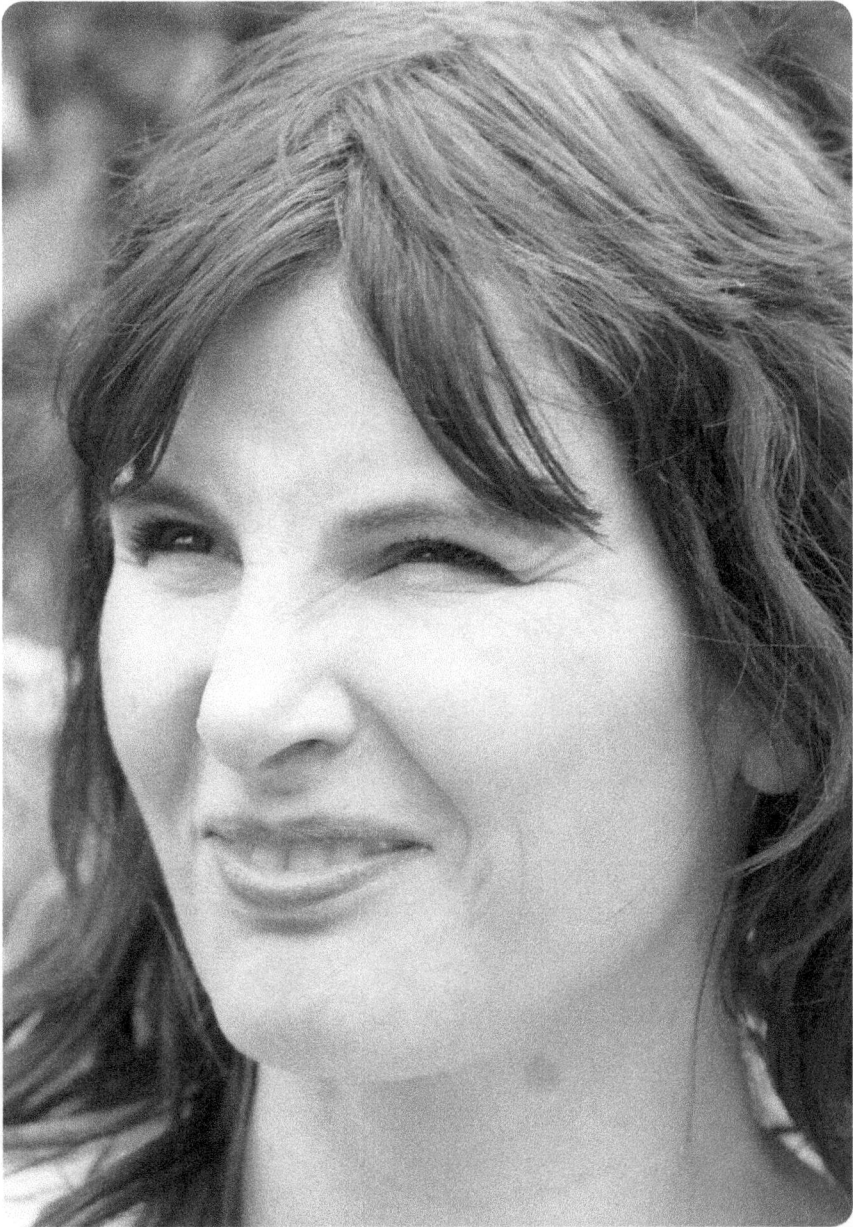

The first time you do the exercise, try out the muscle... the levator labii moves the cheeks straight up towards the eyes, making this expression.

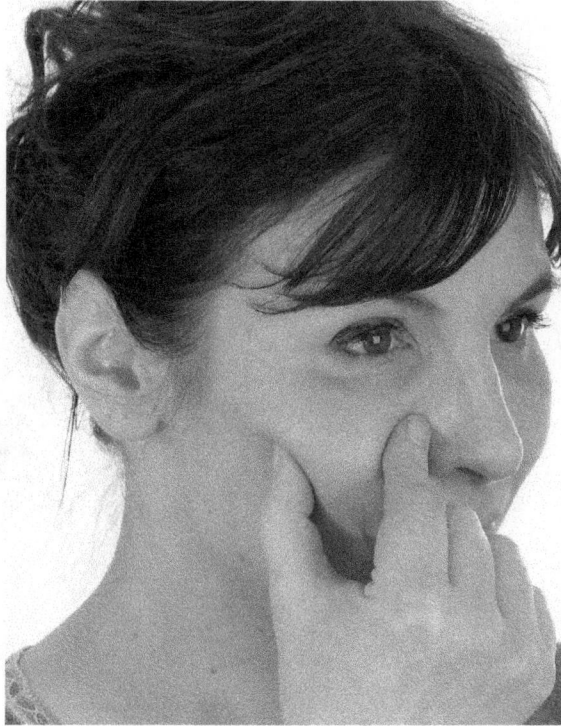

1. Using whatever grip is most comfortable, pinch a chunk of flesh on each cheek alongside the nose, under the eye. Try to grasp as much flesh as possible.

2. Now use the muscle to lift the cheeks straight up toward the centre of the eye.

3. Repeat 20 times, saying each time...

"Delighted to see you"

Checklist

* Grasp as big a chunk of flesh as possible, using any grip you like.

* If you find your grip slipping, you can press the fingers into the face to stabilise them.

* Allow the fingers to 'give' a little so that the muscle can move (as opposed to merely being tensed).

* You might like to do this exercise a few times when you need to see someone else's point of view, for example, if you need to work with a colleague on a project.

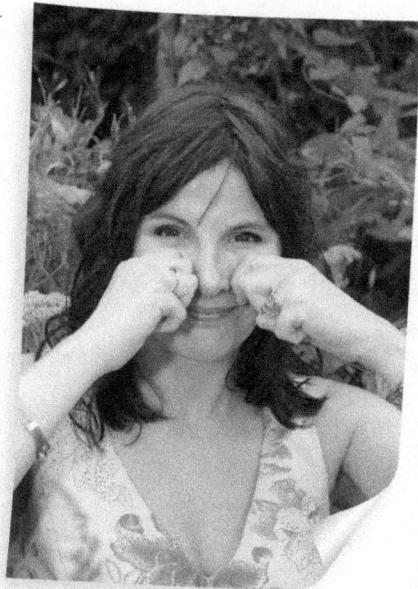

* There are few side-effects in the early days of doing this exercise.

Exercise 2
Lift cheeks 2

Type. A structural exercise.

Muscle. Zygomaticus minor.

Result. Lifts midface up and outward towards the temple.

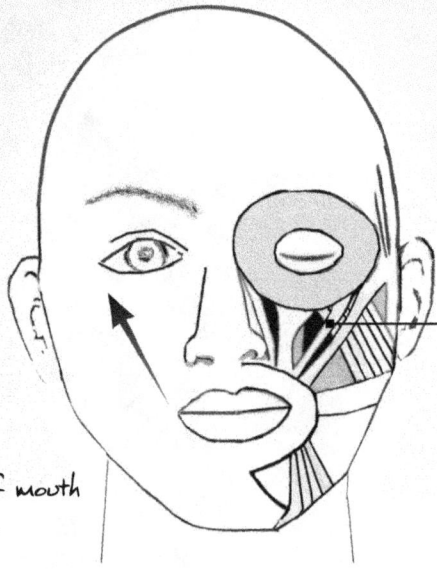

zygomaticus minor

Lifts corners of mouth towards temple.

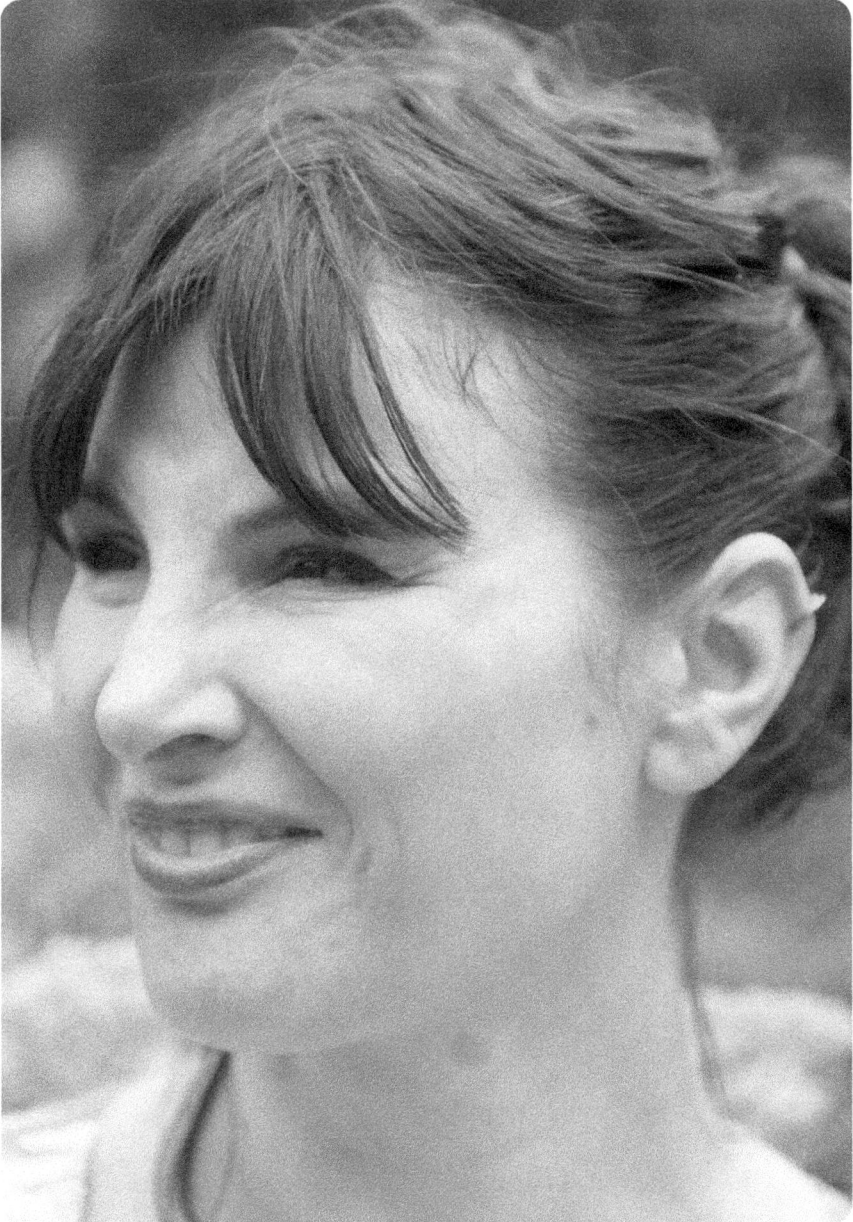

The first time you do the exercise, try out the muscle without using the hands... the zygomaticus minor moves the corners of the mouth up and outward towards the corner of the eye, making this expression.

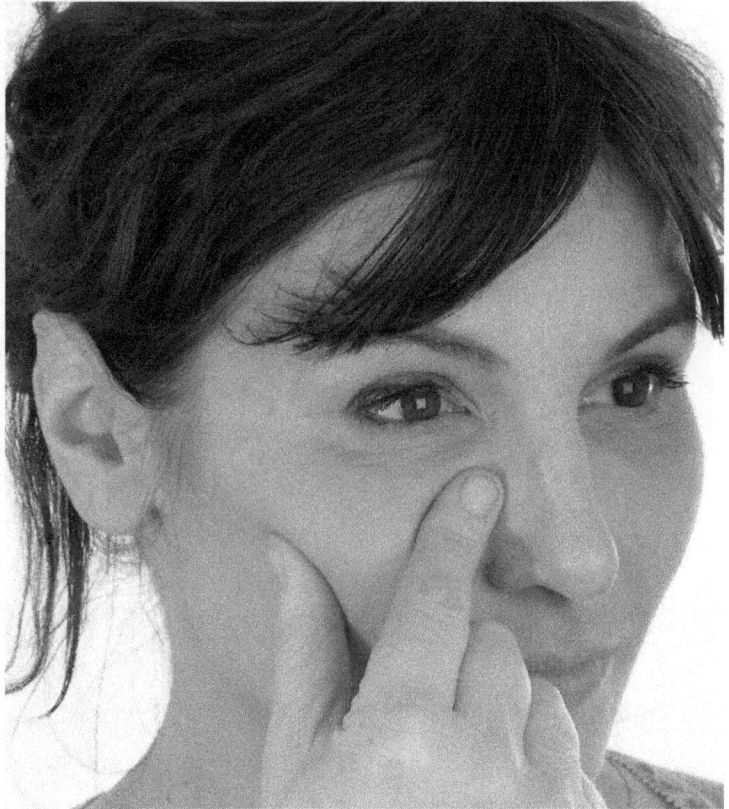

1. Grasp as much flesh as you can along the diagonal from the corner of your mouth to your temple.

2. Now move the corners of the mouth towards the temples.

3. Repeat 20 times, saying each time....

"Delighted to see you"

Checklist

* As with exercise one, any grip, big chunk of flesh.

* Again, press fingers into the face if they slip.

* Allow the fingers to 'give' a little as the muscle moves.

* And once again, it helps get you in the frame of mind to collaborate or cooperate.

* And few side-effects to this exercise, either.

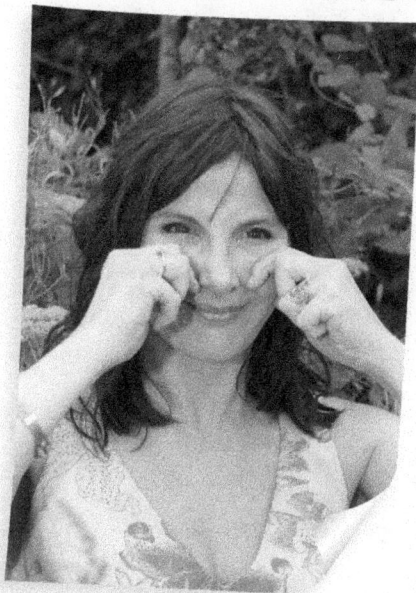

Exercise 3
Happy smile

Type.   A structural exercise.

Muscle.   Zygomaticus major.

Result.   Lifts midface up and outward over the cheekbone
           area.

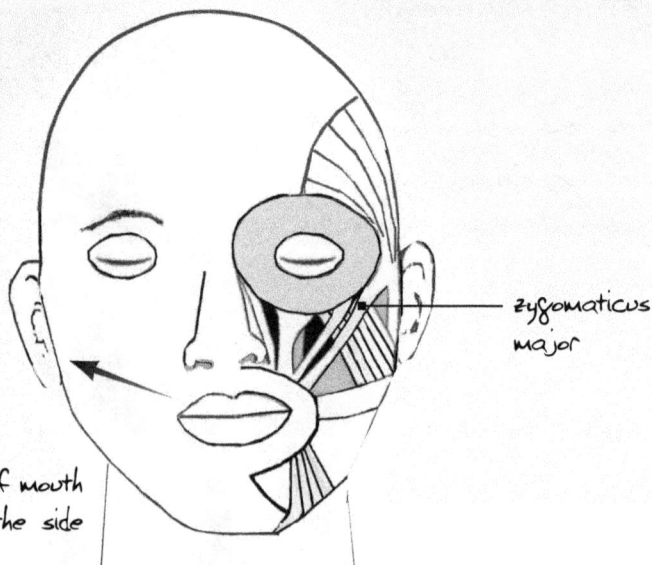

zygomaticus
major

Draws corners of mouth
straight out to the side
(lips apart).

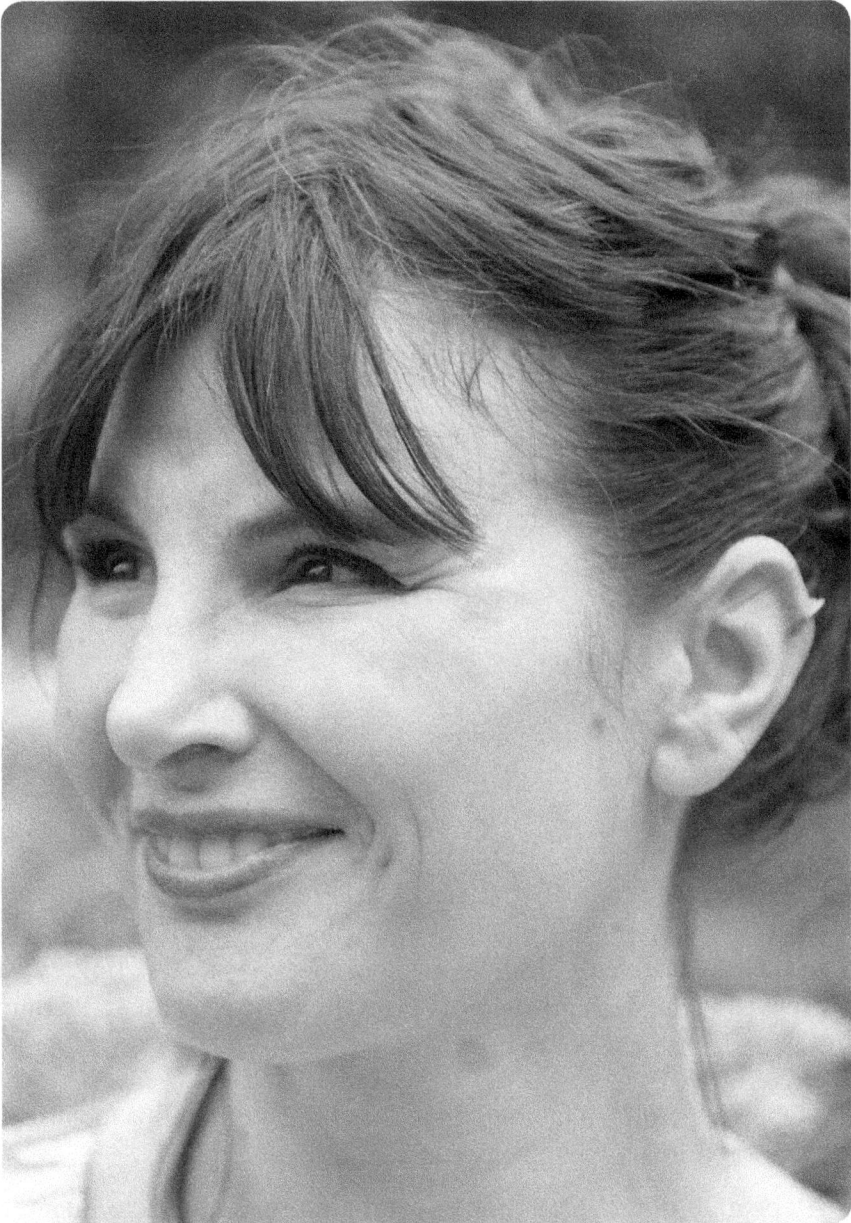

Again, you can try out the muscle without using the hands... the zygo-maticus major moves the corners of the mouth outwards towards the earlobes, making this expression.

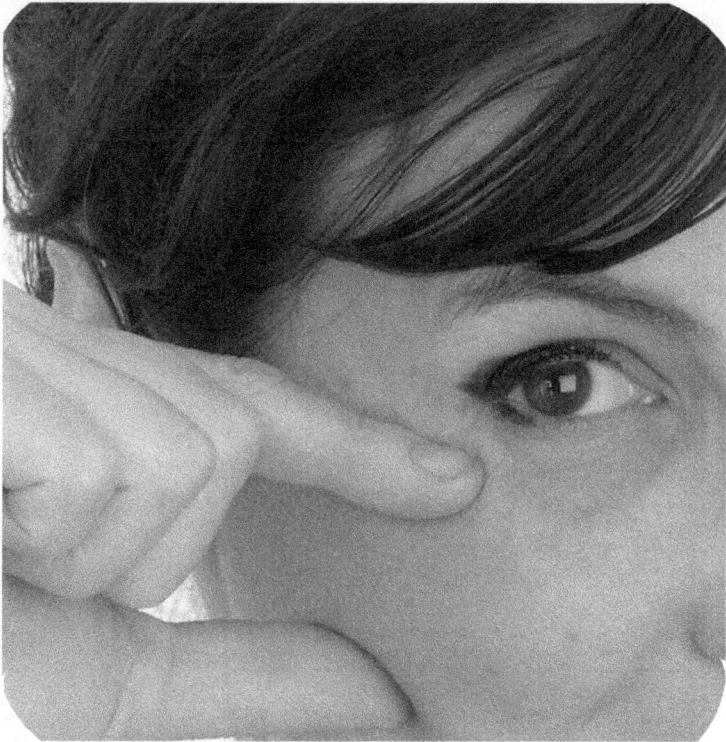

Fingers are on
outer area of cheekbone,
thumb is directly beneath
them, low on the
cheek

1. Grasp a chunk of flesh along the cheekbone…the fingers are pressing the flesh downwards from the eye socket area, the thumb is under the cheek bone.

2. Open the mouth a bit and move the corners of the lips towards the earlobes in a wide, glorious smile.

3. Repeat 20 times, each time encouraging the muscles to make the movement by saying.....

"It's wonderful to feel happy"

Checklist

* Any grip, nice big chunk of flesh, pressing fingers into face.

* Smile right out to the sides as hard as you can.

* Do this exercise to chase away the blues, or just because you feel like being happy.

* Again, few side-effects.

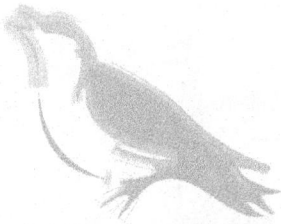

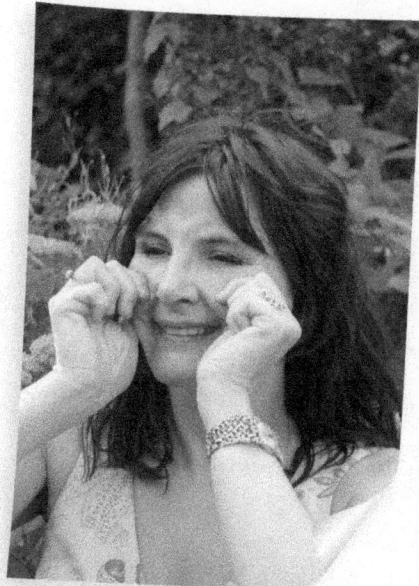

Exercise 4
Laughter

Type. A structural exercise.

Muscle. Risorius.

Result. Draws the face outward from where it has moved downward/inward with age. Sculpts cheekbone area.

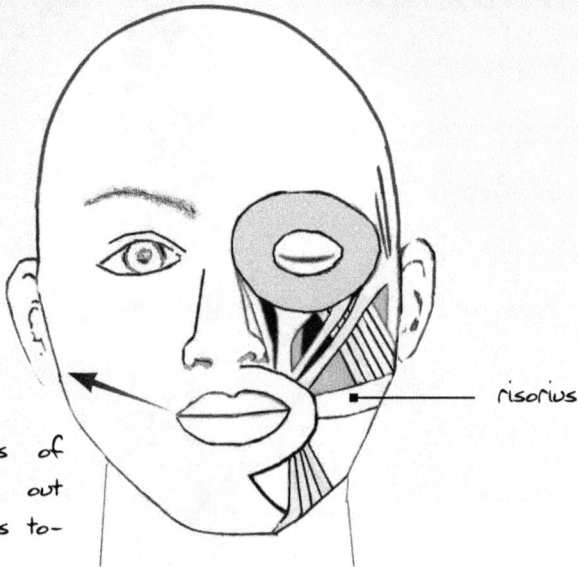

Draws corners of mouth straight out to the side (lips together).

risorius

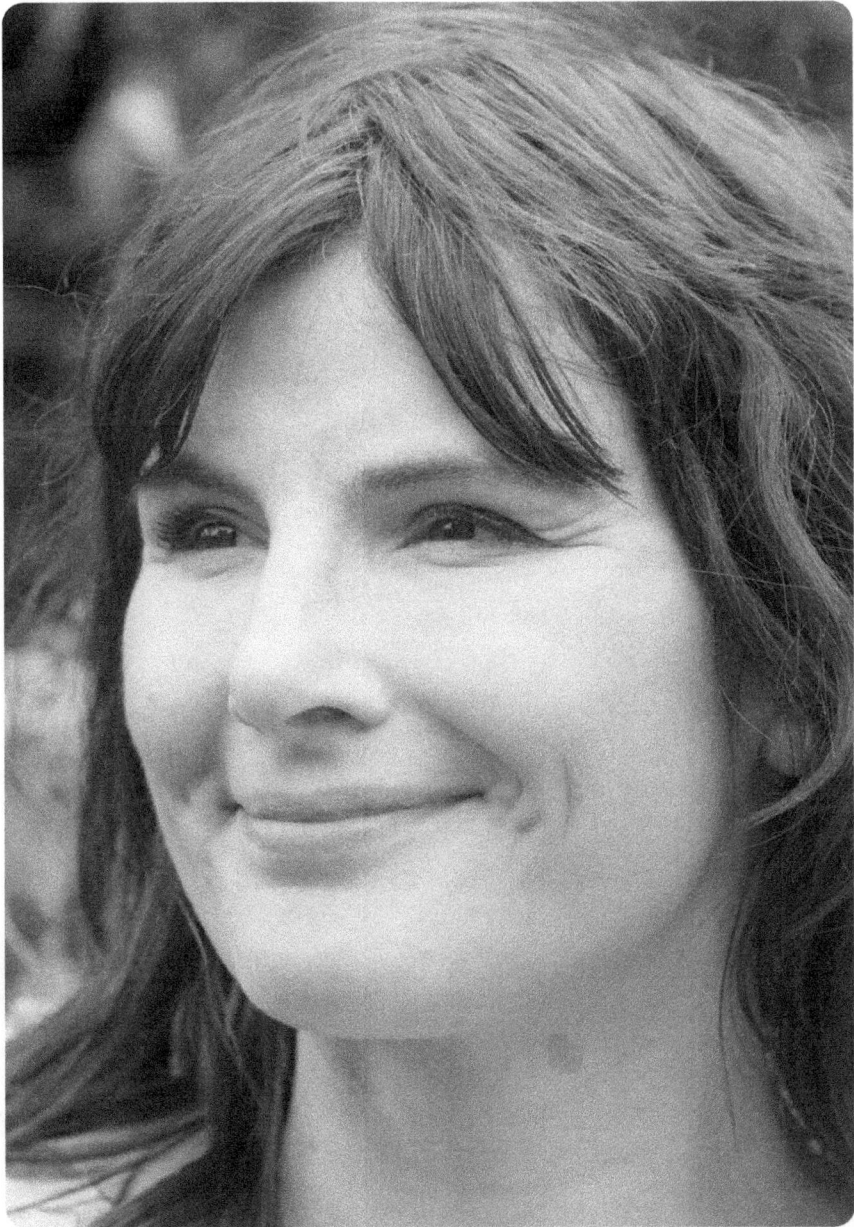

Once again, it's helpful to try out the muscle without using the hands...
the risorius moves the corners of the mouth outwards towards the earlobes, keeping the lips together and making this expression.

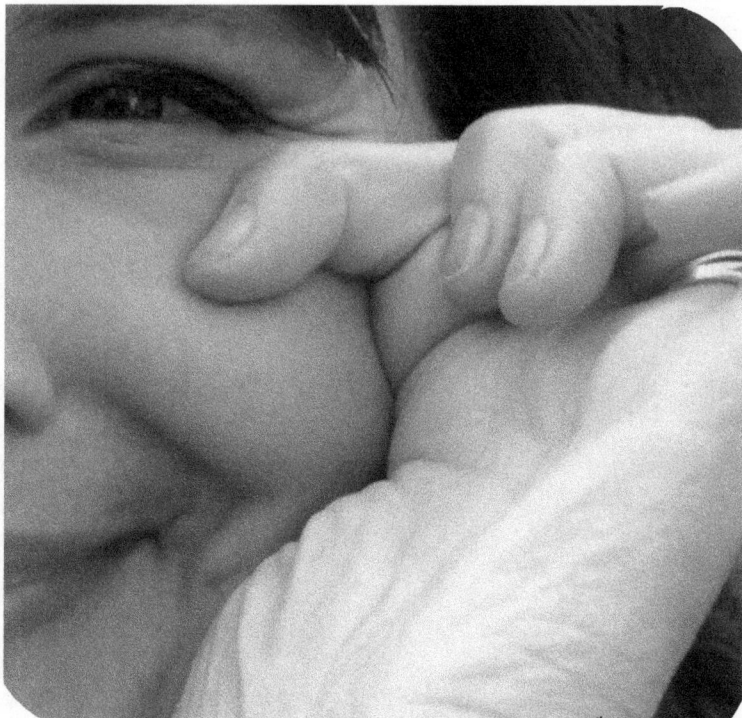

Fingers are on
outer area of cheekbone,
thumb is directly beneath
them, low on the cheek

1. Grasp the face in exactly the same position as for the exercise before this one.

2. Press the lips together firmly as you move the corners of your mouth straight out towards the earlobes, as if you're suppressing a laugh. Try to keep the corners of the mouth against the back teeth.

3. Repeat 20 times, each time saying to yourself.....

66   I love to laugh"

Checklist

* Any grip, nice big chunk of flesh, pressing fingers into face.

* Smile right out to the sides as hard as you can, but press your lips together.

* You can make yourself laugh with this exercise, if you smile widely enough!

* As with most of the struc-tural exercises, there are few side-effects from performing 'laughter'.

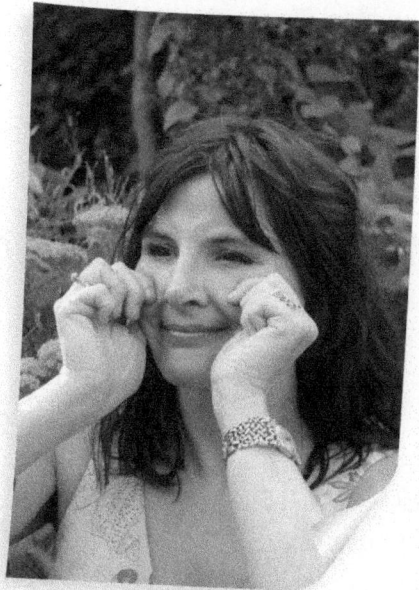

Exercise 5
Sexy beast

Type. A structural exercise.

Muscle. Caninus.

Result. Lifts midface vertically. In particular, lifts out lines nose-mouth.

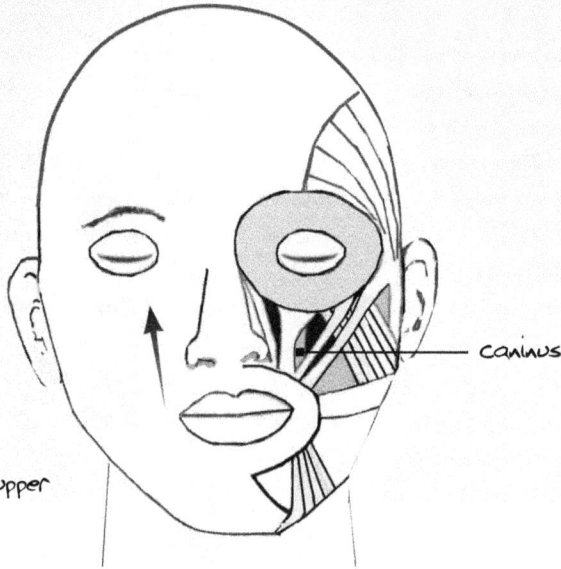

Lift slopes of upper lip straight up.

Caninus

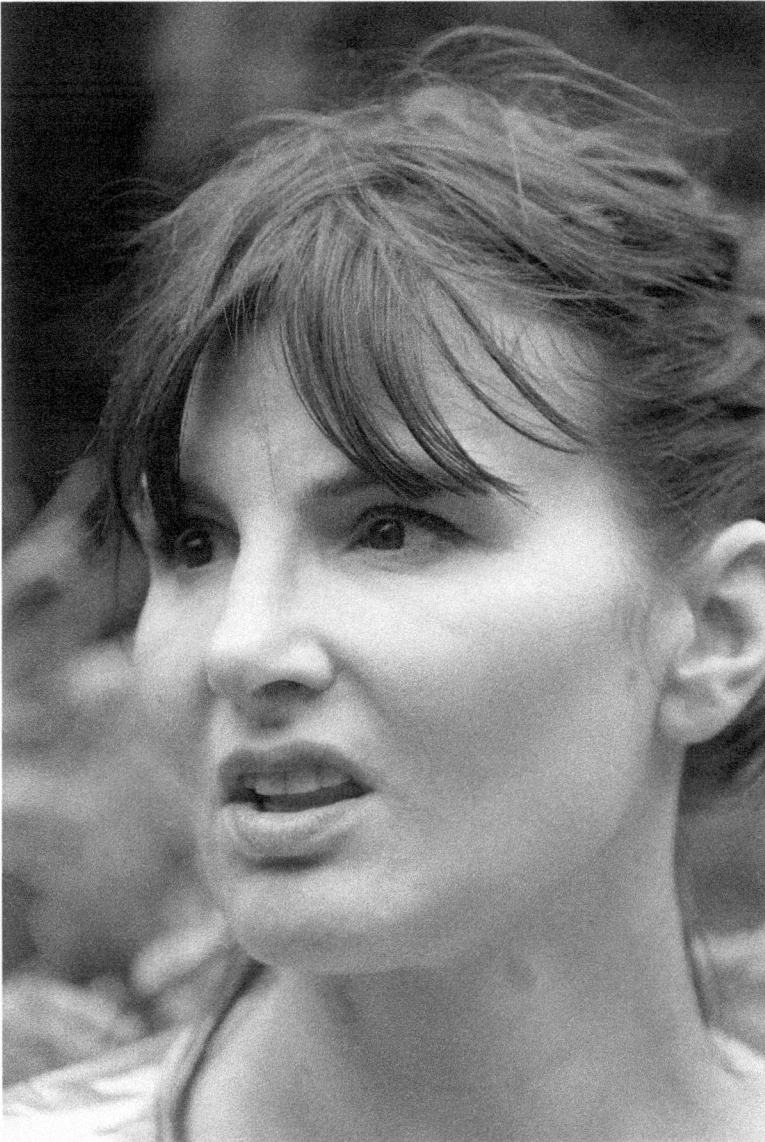

The first time you do the exercise, try out the muscle without using the hands... the caninus pulls a large central area of the lip straight upwards, making this expression.

69

One or two
fingers above bow of lip,
thumb wide on lower
face.

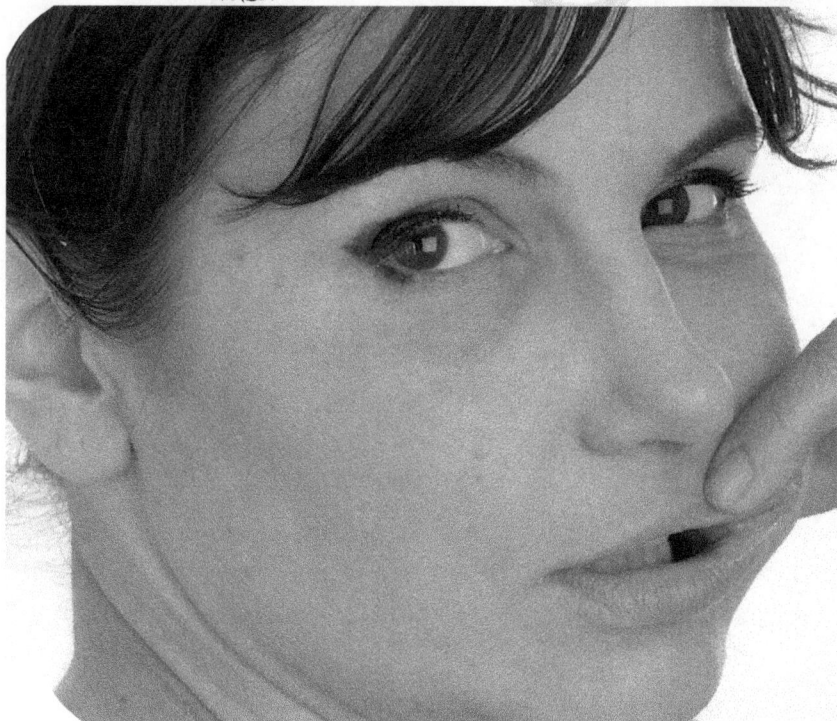

1. Pinch a chunk of flesh either side of the upper lip. The crease from nose to mouth will be amongst the flesh you grasp.

2. Pull the flesh away from the face.

3. Try to curl the upper lip as high as possible and show your teeth in a ferocious snarl.

4. Do this 20 times, saying either...

"You are so sexy", or "I will ROAR"

Checklist

* It can be tricky at first to grasp the area of flesh you need for "Sexy Beast", so you may like to begin by exercising one side at a time.

* A lot of people report that they're not 'feeling' the caninus muscle when they begin (I couldn't feel mine!). It's good to keep going anyway, and you feel it sooner or later. The exercise seems to work the muscle whether you feel it or not, so take heart.

When you get more advanced, pull the flesh outwards, away from the face. The extra stretch does good things for the skin.

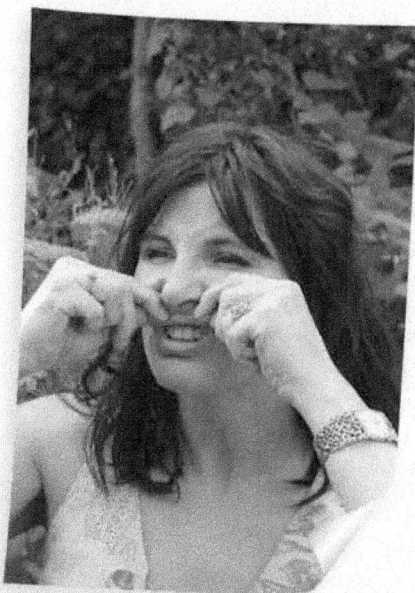

Again, few side-effects.

71

Day two exercises

The first two exercises are designed to sculpt the face.

that is, to encourage the flesh to hug the bone

structure. Most people would welcome a sharper

jawline, but a very sculpted cheek might not be so desirable.

The later exercises are for spot-training, for improving the look

and feel of small local areas of the face.

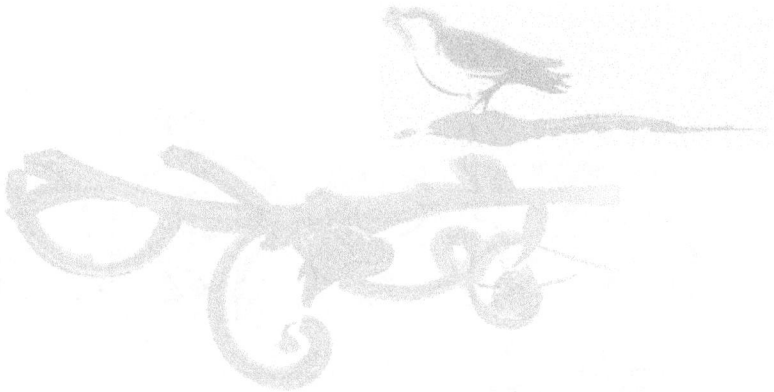

Exercise 6
Crush

Type. A sculpting exercise ie pulls on area of flesh towards the bne structure.

Muscle. Buccinator

Result. Short-term, pulls lower cheeks in dramatically towards the back teeth. Long-term, thickens fleshy area of cheek.

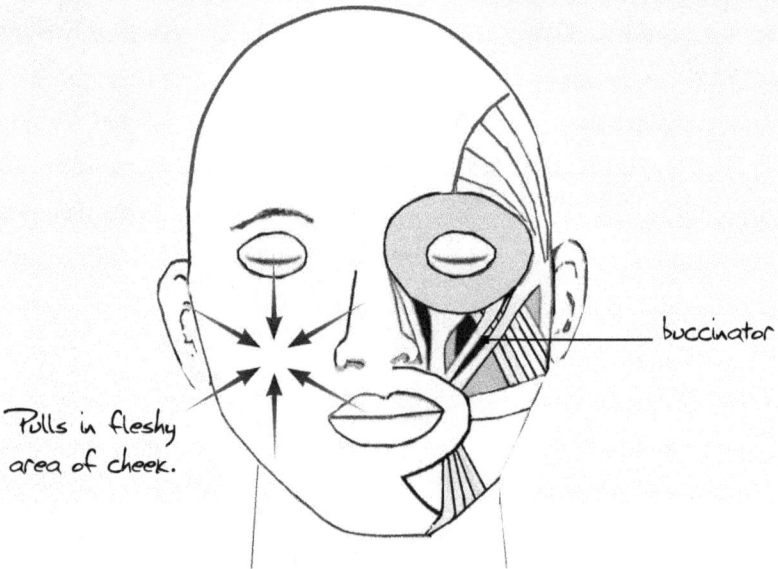

Pulls in fleshy area of cheek.

buccinator

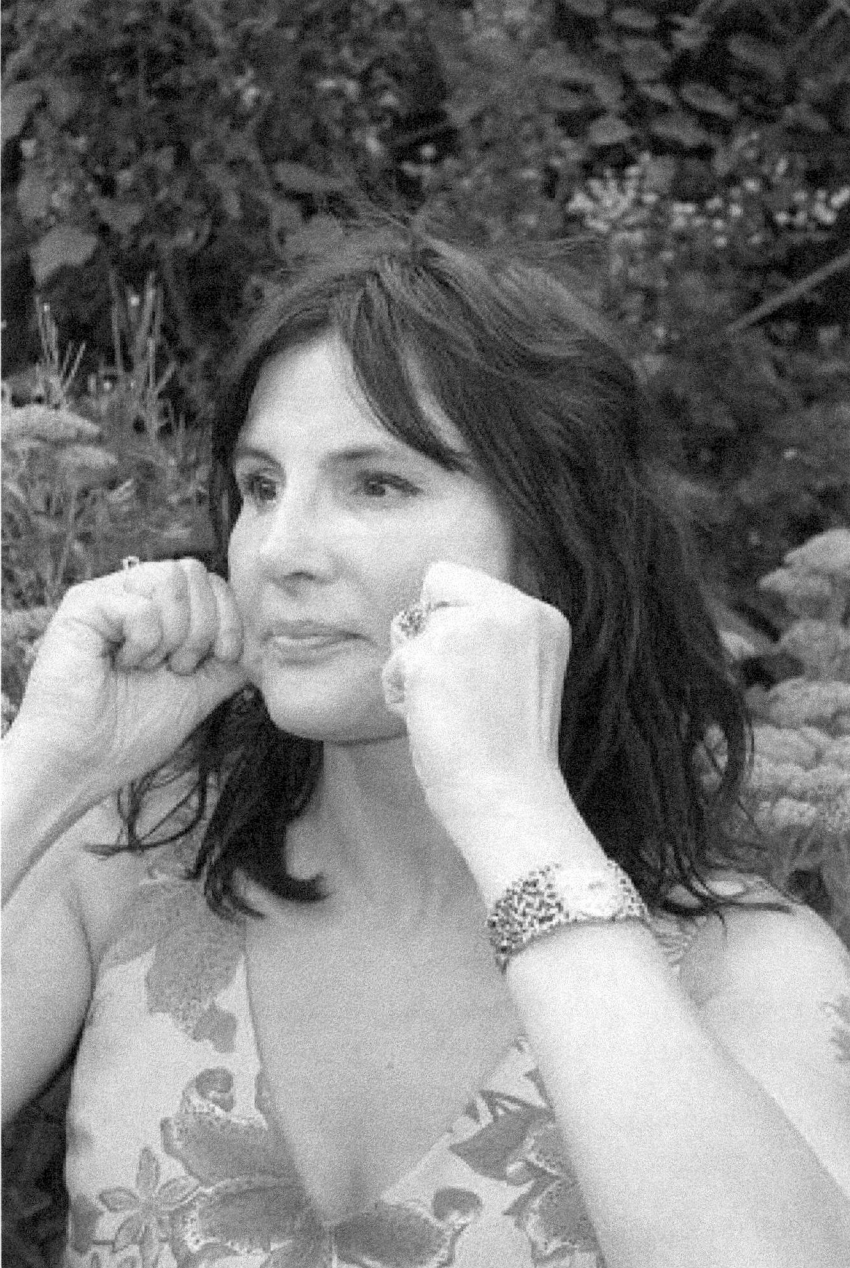

The first time you do the exercise, try out the muscle without using the hands... the buccinator pulls the fleshy parts of the cheek in against the teeth.

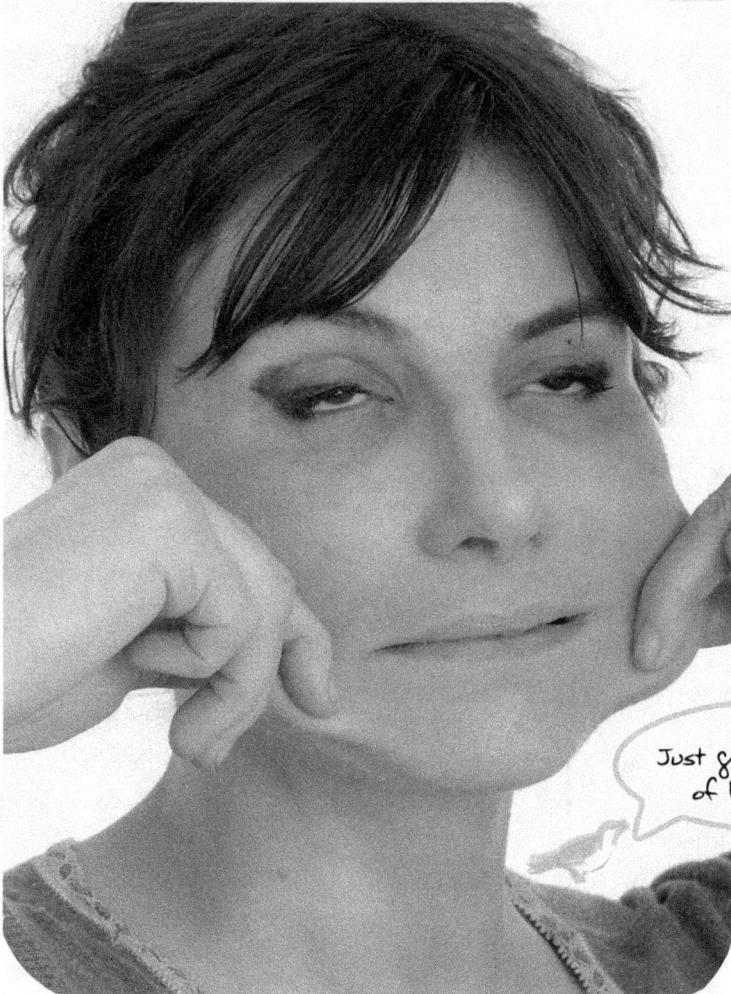

Just grab fleshy area of lower cheek.

1. Put the thumb at the back of the fleshy part of the cheek, under the outer part of the cheekbone.

2. Use the fingertips or side of the finger to pinch as much flesh as you can.

3. Pull this chunk of flesh away from the face.

4. Use the cheek muscles to pull the flesh back to the face. Repeat 20 times. Count to ten each time you repeat this exercise, and imagine crushing fruit with your cheeks.

Note

This exercise will pull the cheeks in dramatically in a very short time. You won't lose any facial fat from doing this exercise, but it's advisable to avoid it if you want to keep your face looking full and plump, as it can take a long time to get through the 'sucked in' stage where the muscle is tightly against the back teeth and begin to to build the area. If you stop doing the exercise, the cheeks will gradually relax again, but again, this can take some time.

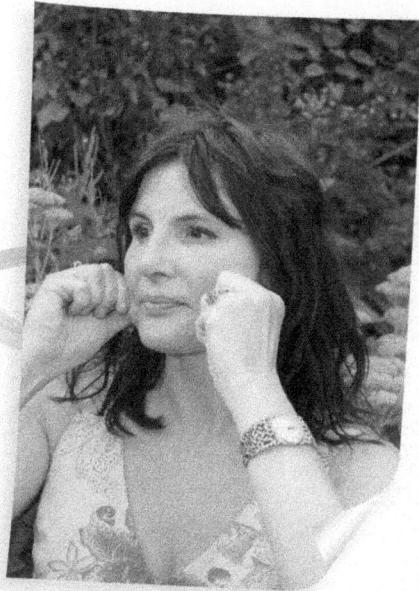

Exercise 7
Long neck

Type. A structural exercise.

Muscle. Platysma.

Result. Firms and sculpts entire jaw/throat area.

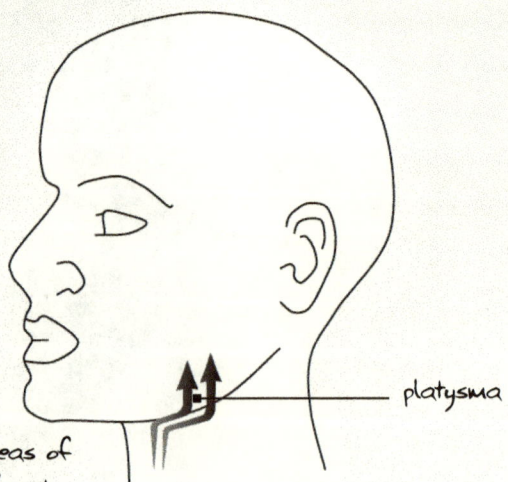

platysma

Pulls in fleshy areas of lower face and throat.

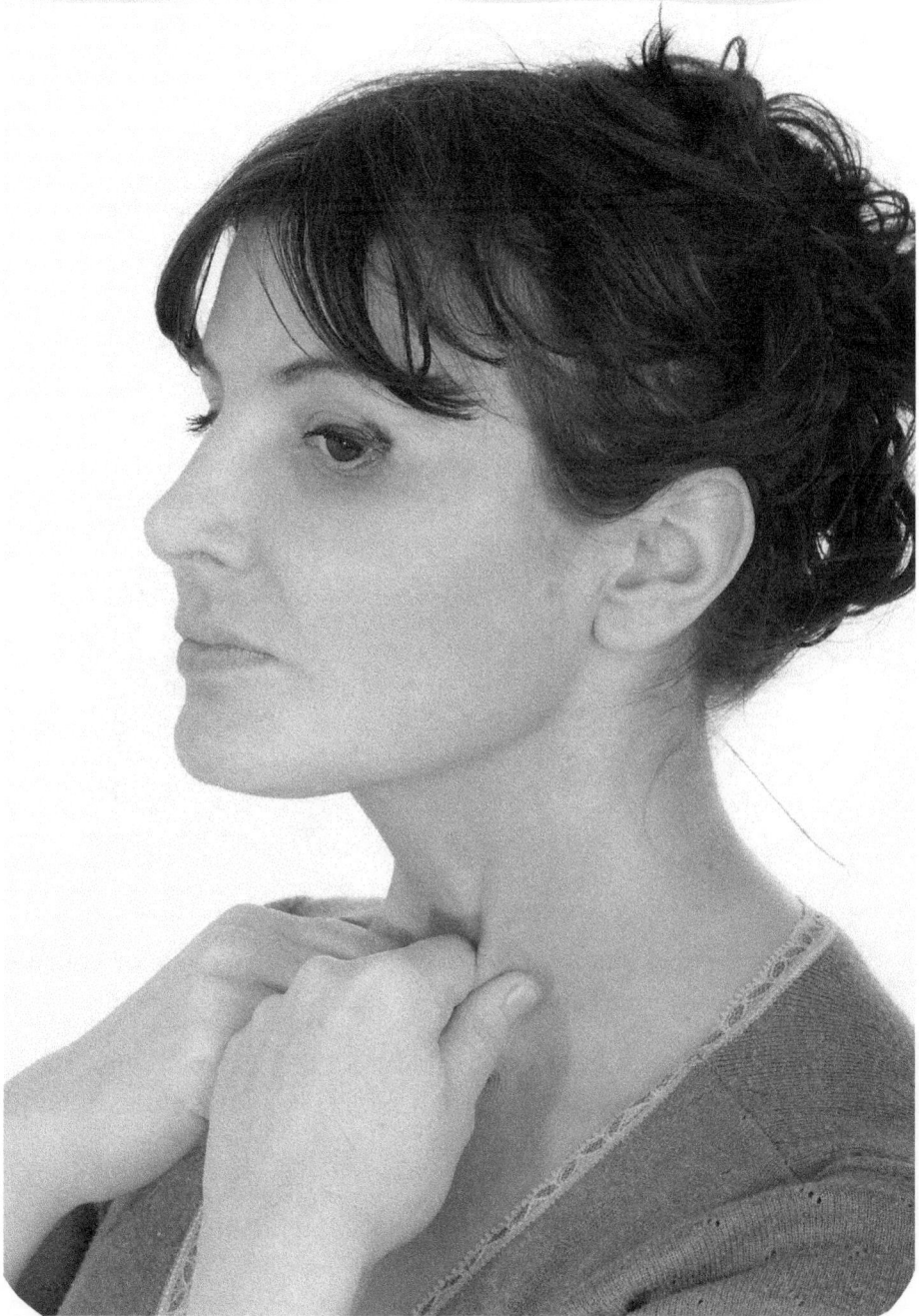

Again, you can try out the muscle without using the hands... the pla tysma produces a little tensing of the jaw as in the picture above.

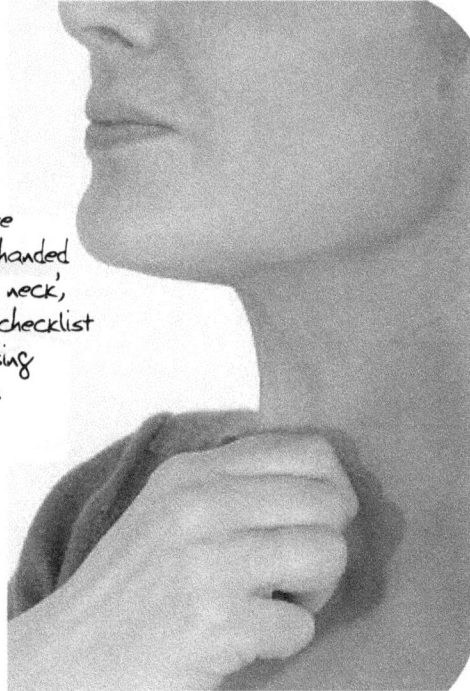

This picture
shows the one-handed
version of 'long neck',
the picture in the checklist
shows me using
both hands

1. Grasp a vertical chunk of flesh (or two, one either side of your windpipe
pull the fleshy areas away from the neck.

2. Tip your head back, open your mouth a little way and tense the
jaw until you feel the flesh move. It may take a little practise, but
in time the muscle will respond.

3. Repeat 20 times, to a slow count of four. Maintain a long, graceful
neck, and stretch the neck further as you contract the muscle. Say,

"long graceful neck"

Checklist

Pull the flesh out and away from the neck as much as you can comfortably manage, to strengthen the skin while you exercise.

If you have trouble 'feeling' the platysma, try turning the corners of the mouth down to get used to feeling where it is. Move on to performing the exercise without doing this when you're

Some people are concerned that the programme includes so few exercises for the neck and add headlifts or other exercises to supplement the day two routine.

The platysma is the only muscle of the neck that pulls the skin up and inwards to the jawbone. Any risidual looseness of the skin will improve over time as it adjusts to the new contour of the neck. Most other exercises will simply build up the neck and

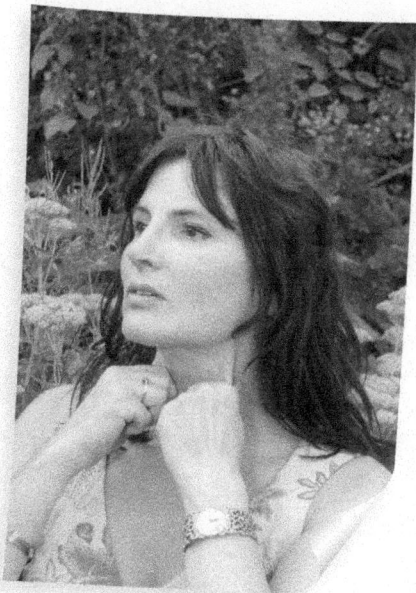

veloped muscles show under the

prove the way the skin lies on

Exercise 8
Wish

Type.   A spot-training exercise.

Muscle.   Orbicularis oculis.

Result.   Firms entire eye area, including lids, undereye area, browbone. Eventually smooths out hollow areas, eliminates lines, wrinkles or baggy areas above or below the eye.

Squeezes
eyes shut.

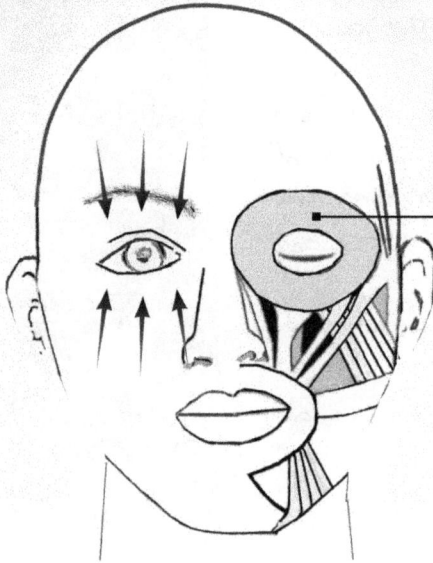

orbicularis oculis

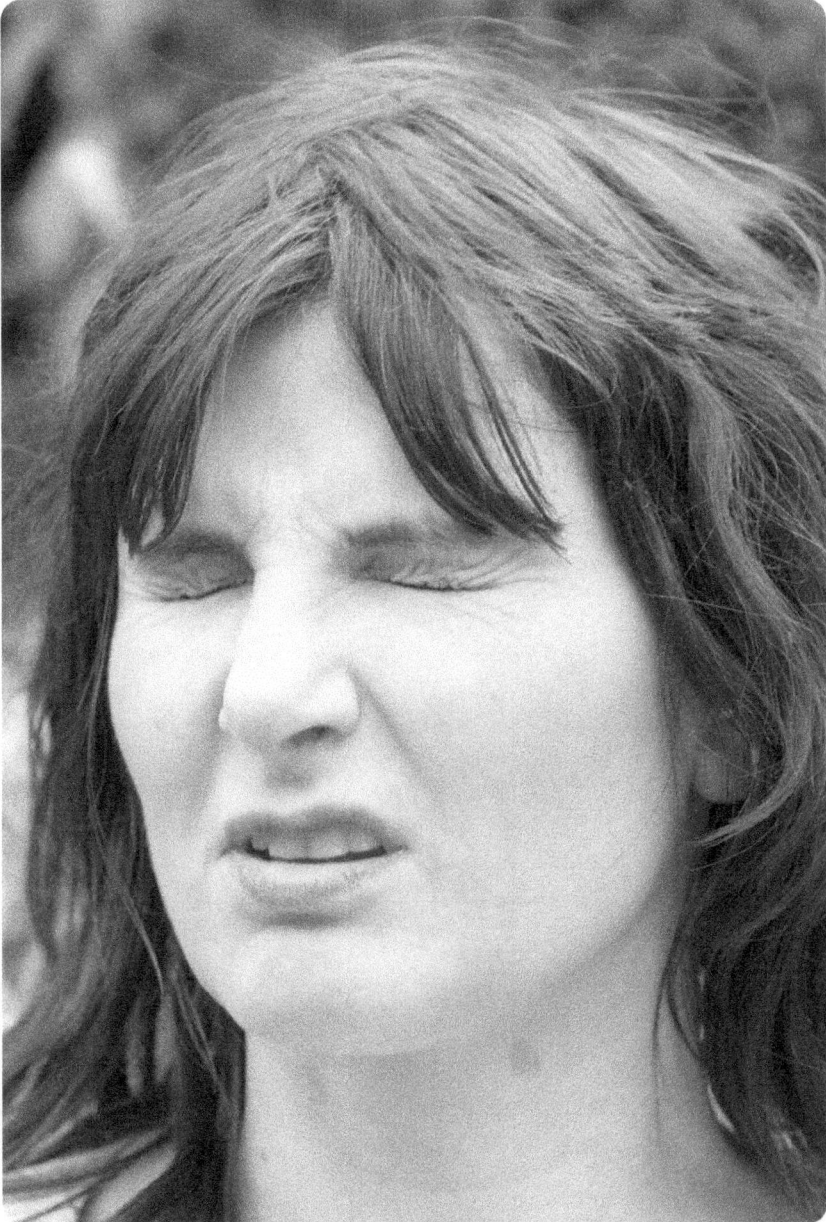

'Wish' is easy expression-wise, but if you're in any doubt, the eyes are squeezed tightly shut, as illustrated here.

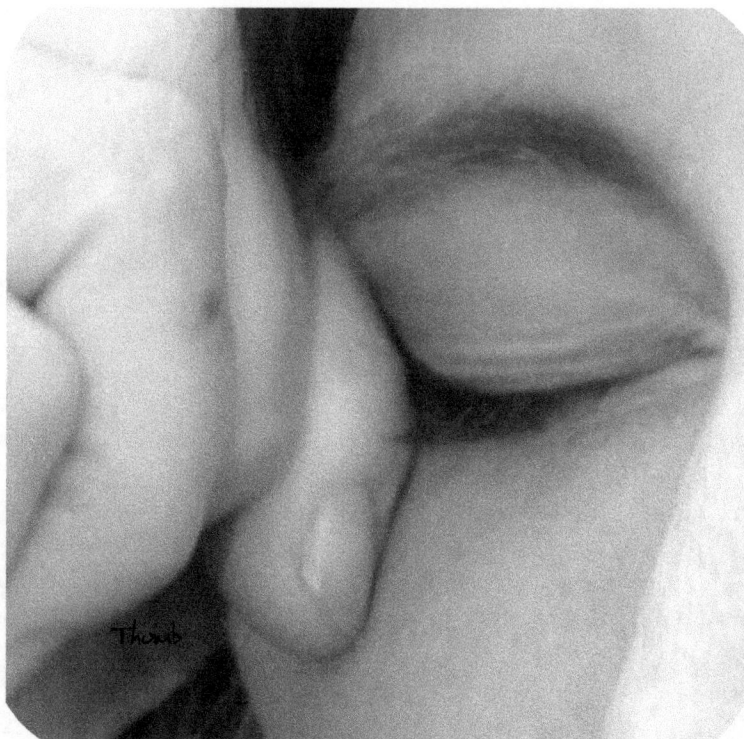

Thumb

1, 2 or 3 fingers
at outer corner of eye,
thumb at temple , pinch as
much skin as you
can.

1. Pinch a chunk of flesh between the outer corner of the eye and the temple. The corner of the eye needs to be anchored by one of your digits.

2. Squeeze eyes tightly shut.

3. Repeat 20 times as rapidly as possible, while ensuring you squeeze the eys as hard as you can.

Checklist

* It's good to make sure both the outer area and the inner (eye-lid) areas of the muscle are engaged, you may like to squint for a moment before you squeeze the eye shut to make sure that you're contracting all the rings of muscle fibre.

* Because the exercise requires you to scrunch the muscle, temporary lines can sometimes appear around the eye after exercise. When the muscle becomes healthy and elastic enough to spring back to its flat resting shape immediately this will stop happening.

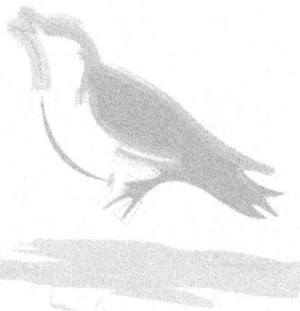

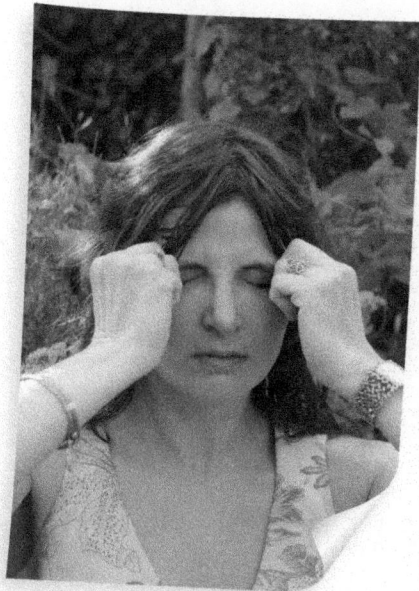

Exercise 9
Lift eyelids

Type. A spot-training exercise.

Muscle. Levator palpebrae.

Result. Widens eyes.

Opens upper
lid of eyes.

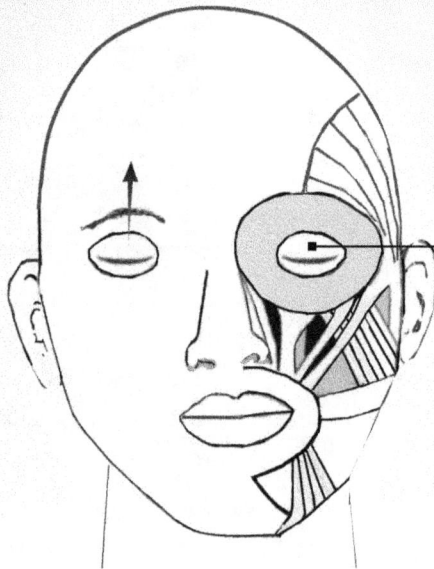

levator palpebrae

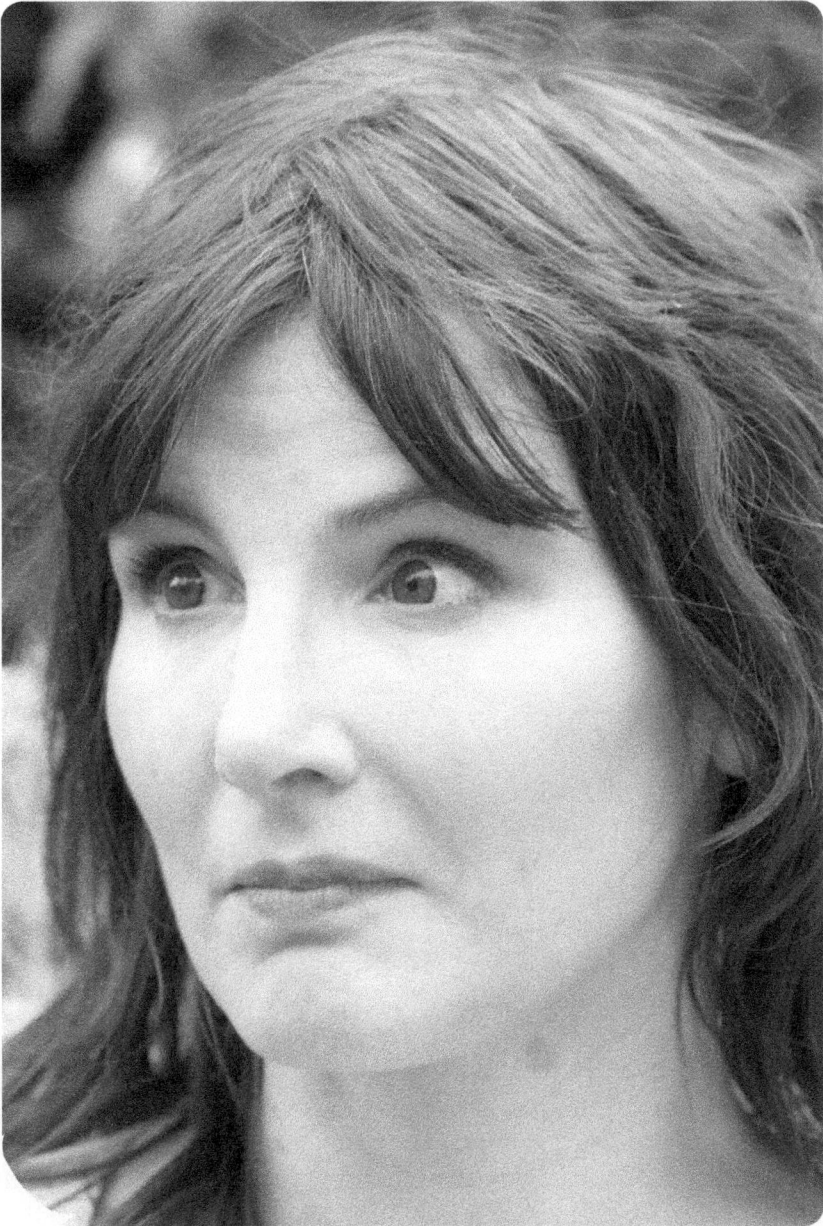

Again, not difficult to recognise the expression... eyes are open as wide as possible, but this muscle is often weak to begin with, keep practising opening your eyes wide whenever you get chance.

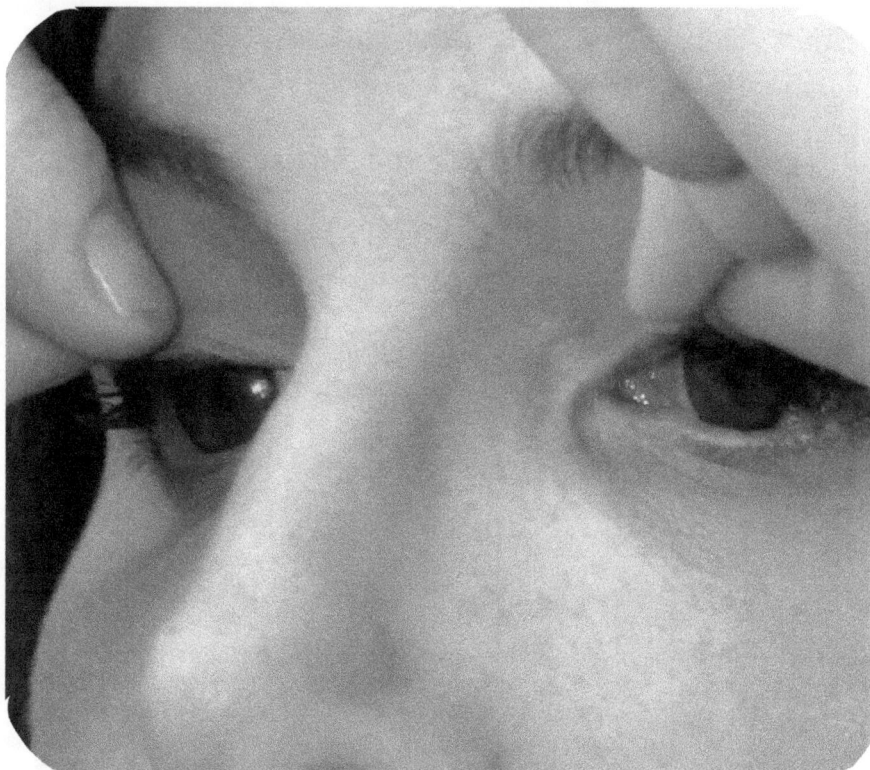

Finger
at inner corner of
eye, thumb at outer corner,
pinch whole eyelid.

1. With the eyes closed, pinch the upper lid from corner to corner between finger and thumb

2. Open the eyes as wide as you can. If you can't open them, relax the fingers a little. Just trying is good.

3. Do it 20 times. To enjoy the feeling of attentiveness, and to make the movement feel easy and natural say,

"There is so much to amaze me"

Checklist

* This exercise allows you to handle and really stretch the skin of the eyelid. Don't be afraid to pull the lid away from the eyeball.

* The levator palpebrae isn't always easy to engage at first, but with very little practice it will strengthen and widen the eye very quickly.

* There should be few side-effects, although the eyes can look tired for a few days if they're overtrained, they soon recover.

* You can use this exercise to prepare you for an occasion where you need to be alert and focussed. It's very effective in helping your concentration.

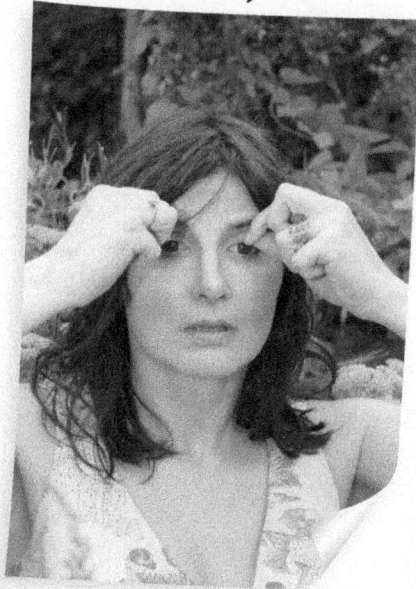

Exercise 10
Kiss

Type.	A spot-training exercise.
Muscle.	Naso-labialis.
Result.	Lifts, firms and significantly thickens upper lip.

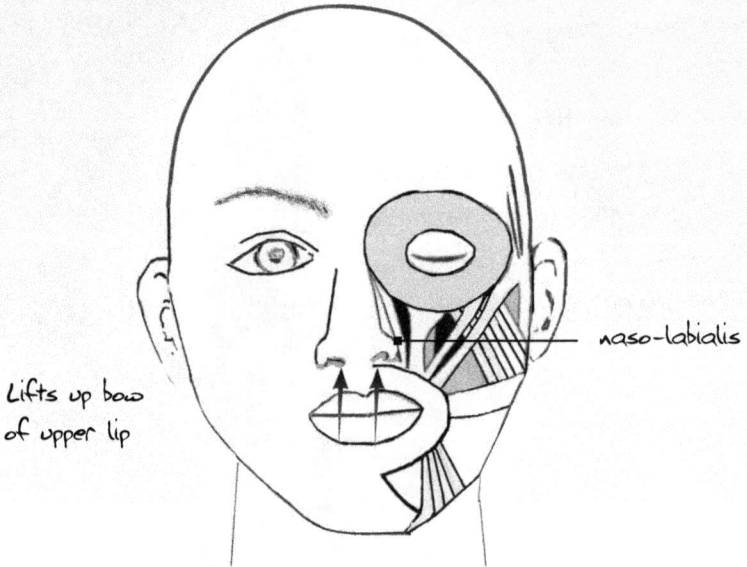

Lifts up bow of upper lip

naso-labialis

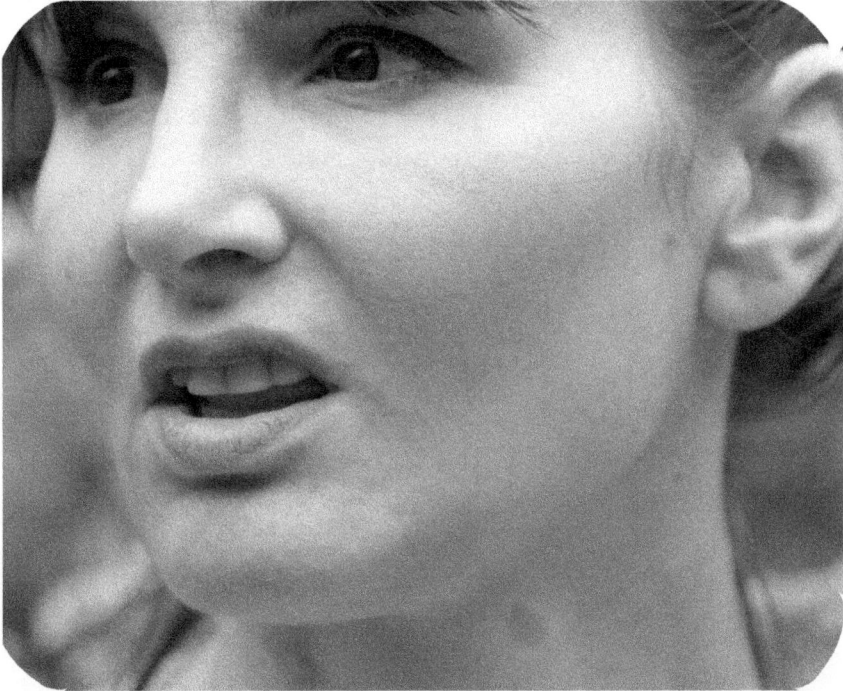

The upper lip lifts, as in the picture, but you may like to try saying 'tch' until the movement comes easily to you.

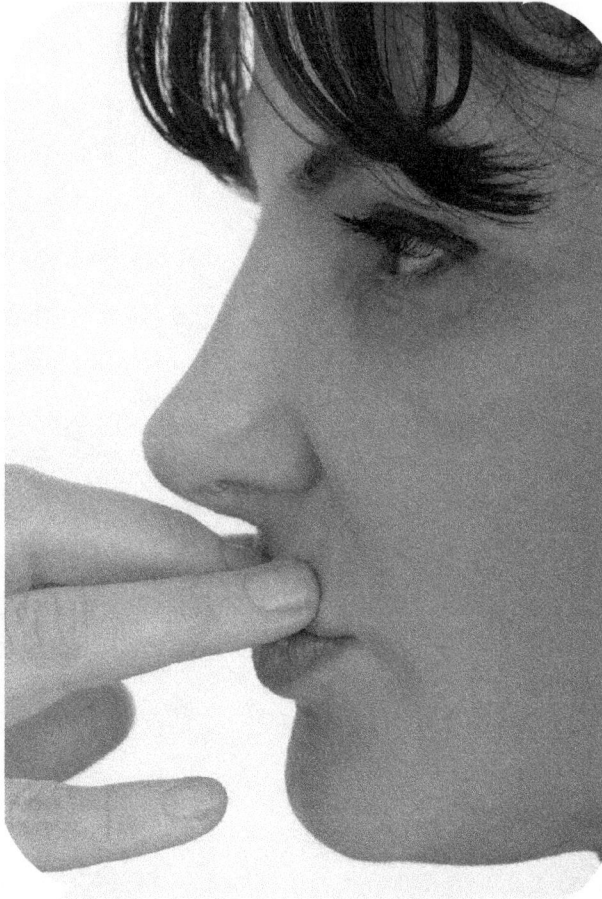

1. Place three fingers of one hand on your upper lip.

2. Use the lip muscle to curl the upper lip outwards up and away from the upper teeth.

3. You can do this exercise any time as it's discreet. You don't hold the finishing position, just keep repeating the movement.

Checklist

* If you can't immediately master the movement, you can feel it by saying the sound 'ch'. Once you know how to move the muscle, though, it feels better to say, 'kiss my mouth'

* Just do this exercise whenever you want to feel gorgeous.

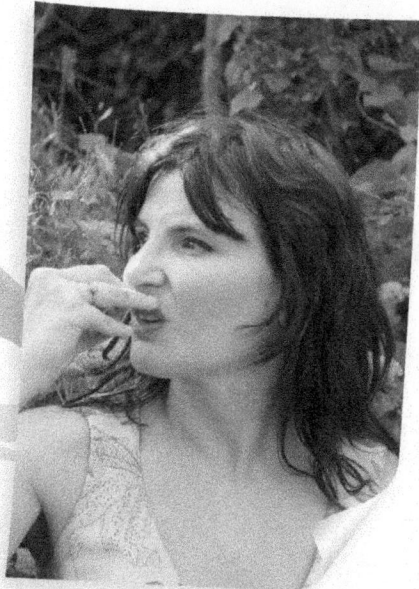

Occasional extras

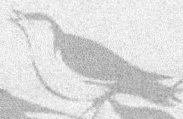

These exercises need to be done rarely, no more often than once every four weeks. The muscles being trained don't directly lift the flesh, and don't benefit from being developed. They just need to be kept firm without encouraging their growth.

Alternative 1
Lift brows

Type. Occasional spot training exercise.

Muscle. Frontalis.

Result. Maintains firm forehead.

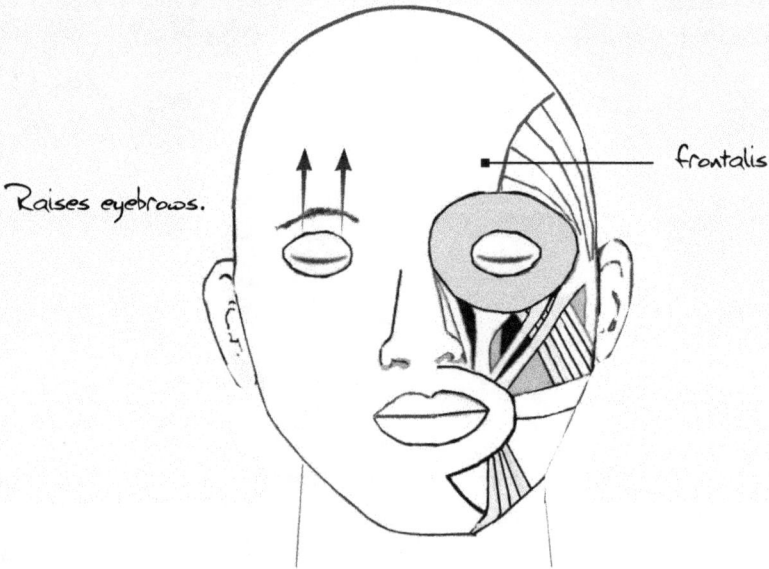

Raises eyebrows.

frontalis

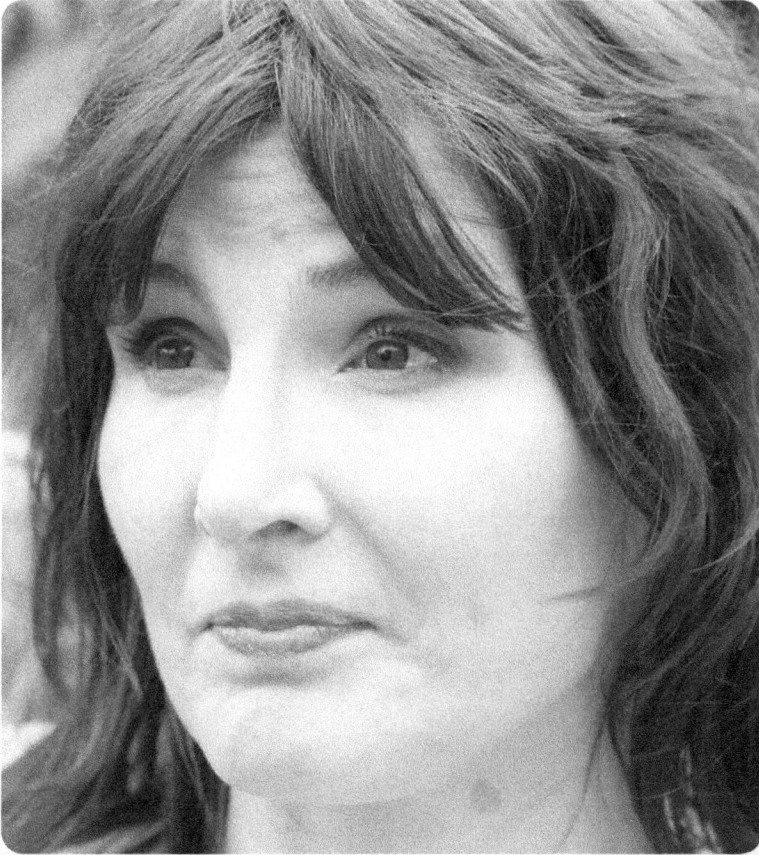

The expression without hands is just raised eyebrows as above.

Note: This is an area I'm divided about. It's important to the scalp, and it's obviously not great if the whole area slides down and droops over the eyes and nose, so it needs some exercise.

But as I explained at the start of this book, the facial muscles lose their ability to snap back to their flat shape and so pull the skin into wrinkles. The frontalis especially will assume its furrowed shape for longer and more extremely the more often you use it, and this increase in furrowing can go on for a long time before the muscle becomes strong and elastic enough to lie flat again. This is why it's in this section instead of one of the others.

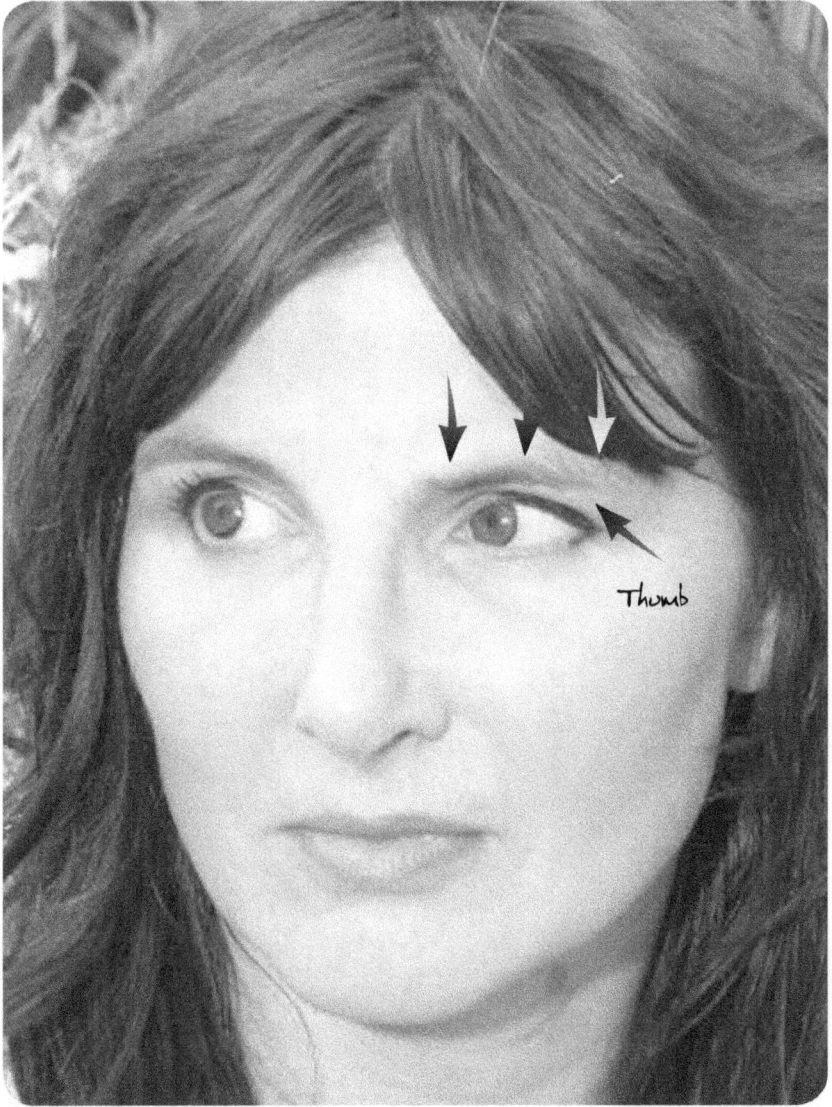

Thumb

1. Grasp a chunk of flesh along the eyebrow and pull it away from the face

2. Raise the eyebrows!

3. Repeat 10 times

Checklist

* Remember to enjoy the stretch as you pull the brows away from the face.

* Contracting a muscle, especially for spot-training exercise will often produce temporary wrinkles. The frontalis especially will assume its furrowed shape for longer and more extremely the more often you use it, and this increase in furrowing can go on for a long time before the frontalis becomes strong and elastic enough to lie flat again, so it's wise to use it only occasionally to avoid the side-effects.

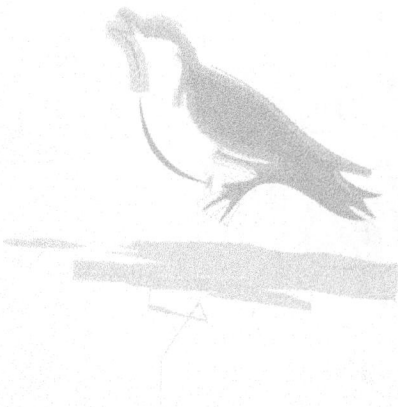

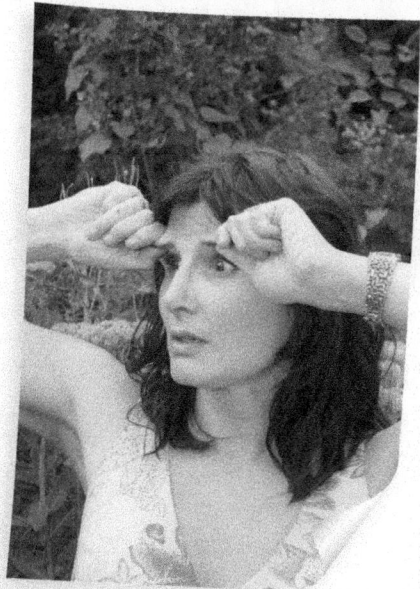

Alternative 2
Central Forehead

Type. Occasional spot training exercise.

Muscle. Procerus.

Result. Maintains firmness in the central, lower area of the forehead and bridge of nose.

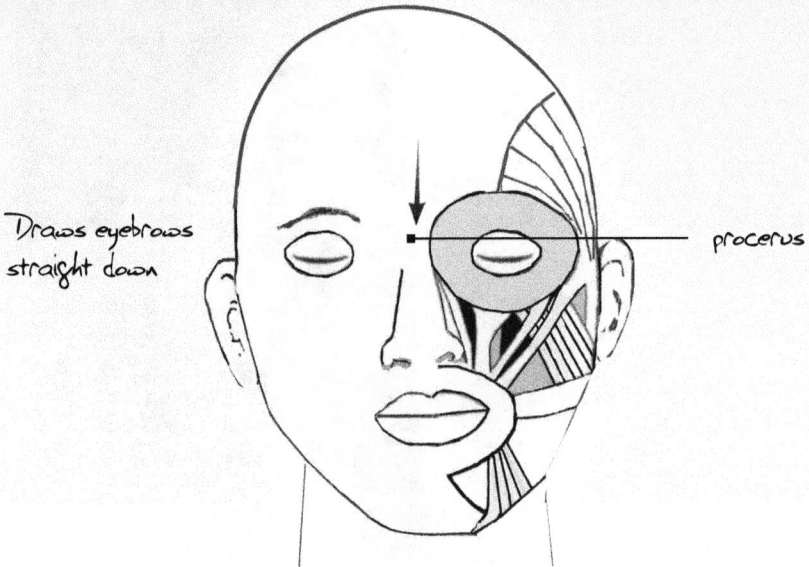

Draws eyebrows straight down

procerus

Sorry to look so unfriendly in some of these pics

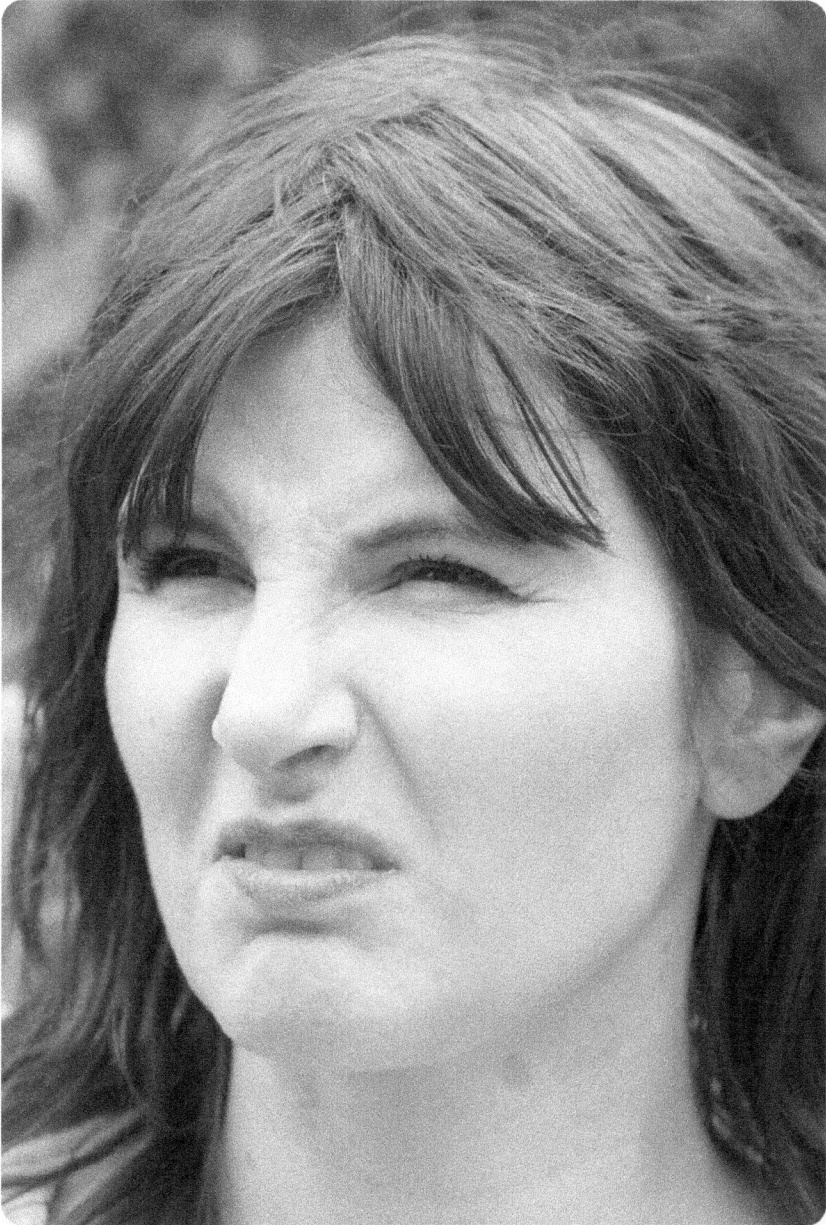

The first time you try this it's sensible to see how the muscle feels without hands. The nose wrinkles and the brow moves straight down as illustrated here.

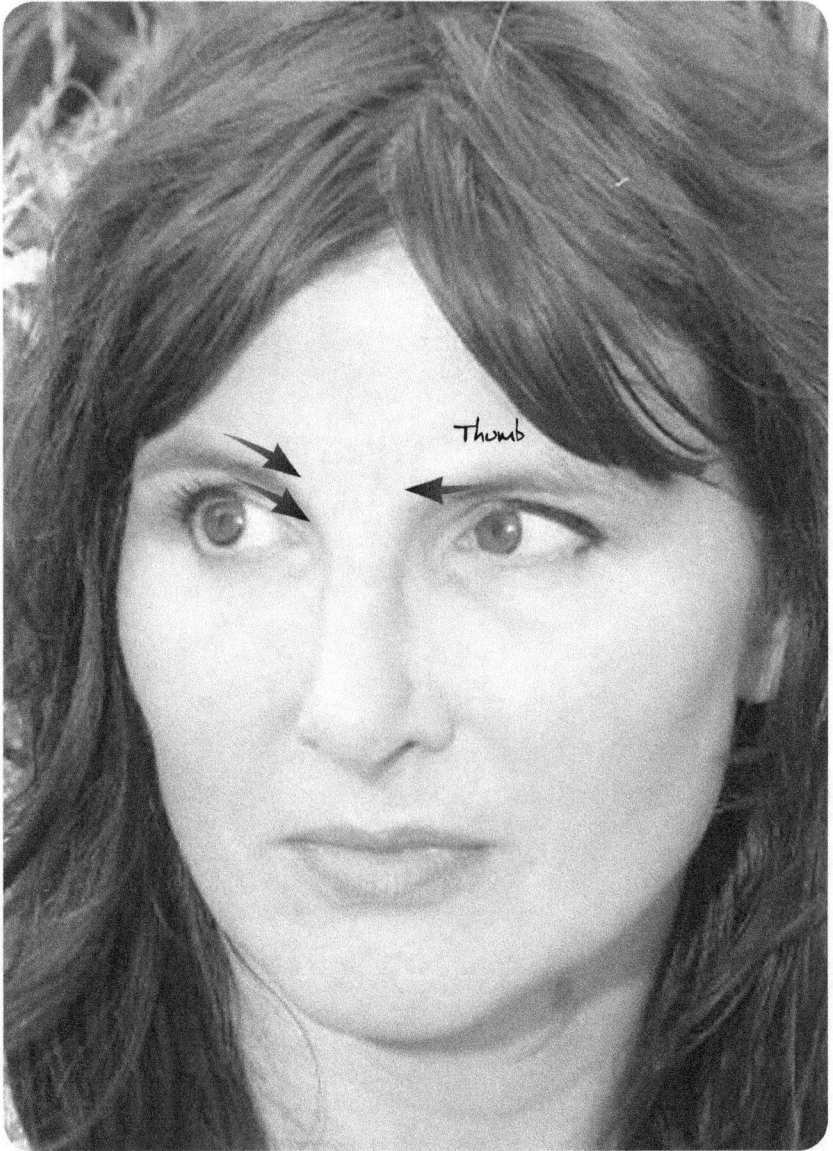

1. Pinch the skin between the brows, above the bridge of the nose.

2. Wrinkle the nose without frowning.

3. Repeat 10 times

Checklist

* Again, pull firmly on the area you grasp so as to benefit the skin as well as the muscle.

* Move the muscle by wrinkling the nose rather than drawing the brows downward.

* When performed occasionally there should be few side-effects to this exercise, but overuse can build the area up and produce a cro-magnon appearance which isn't very feminine. I'd restrict the use of this exercise to once a month at most... it only needs a little attention to keep it firm.

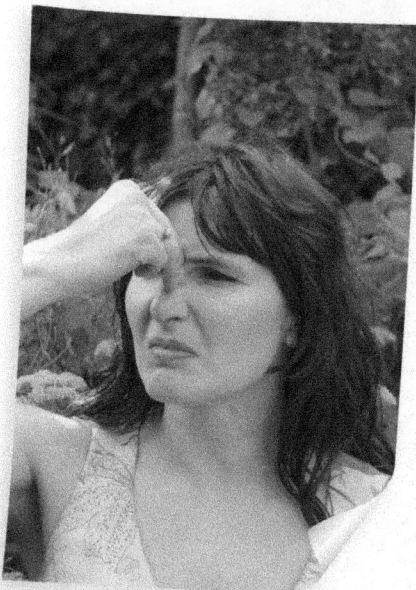

Alternative 3
Head high

Type. Occasional structural exercise.

Muscle. Masseter, temporalis.

Result. Allows you to hold the jaw as you did when young, ie close to the upper jaw.

Both muscles close the jaw.

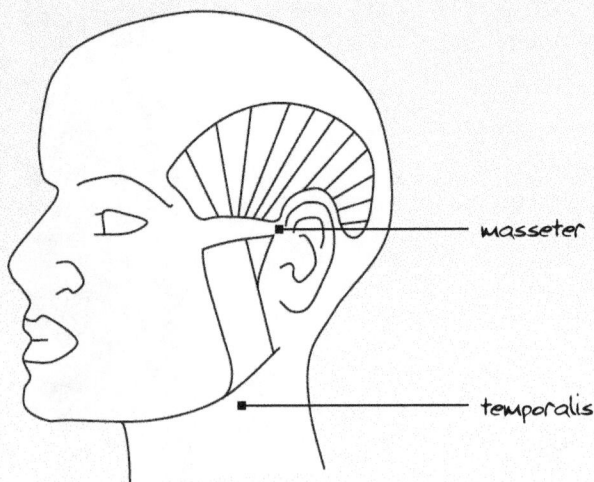

masseter

temporalis

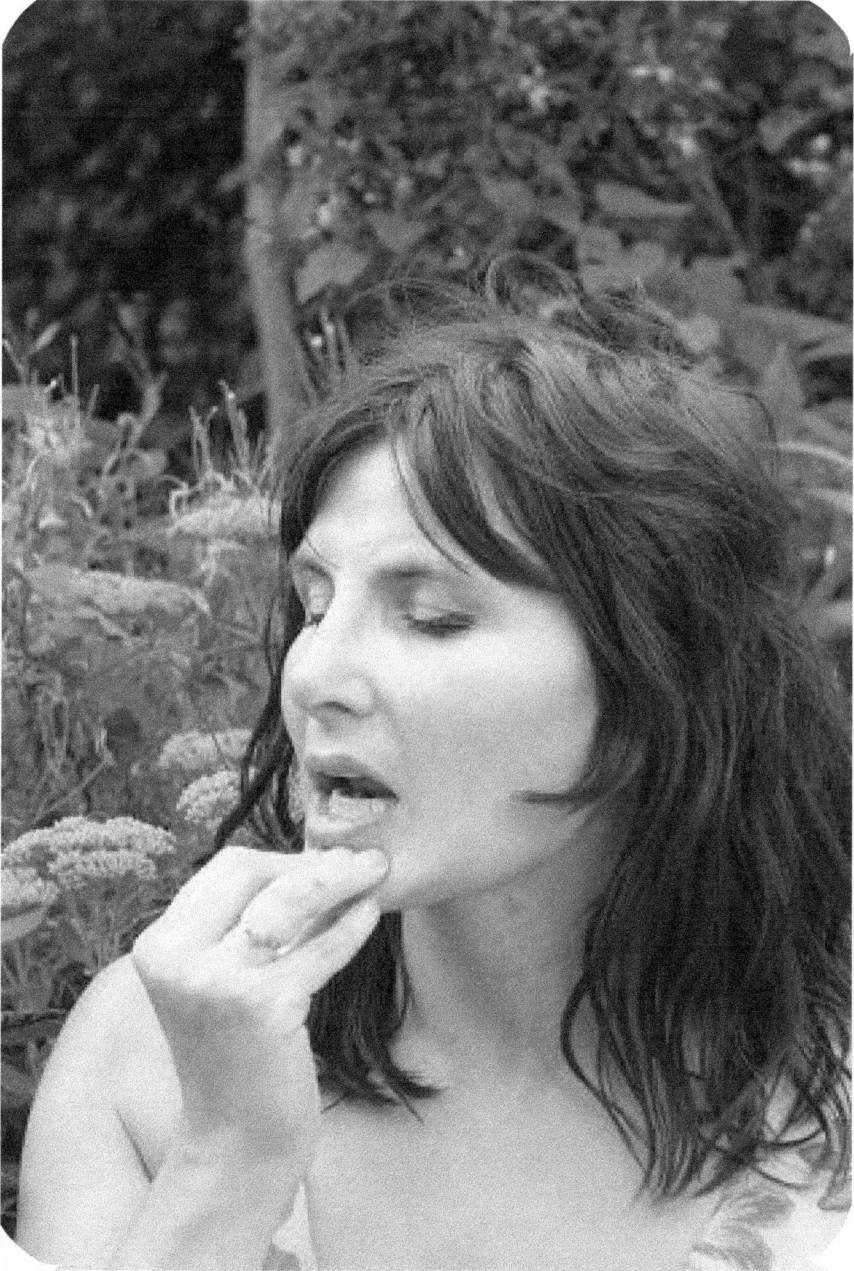

The movement is just opening and closing the mouth

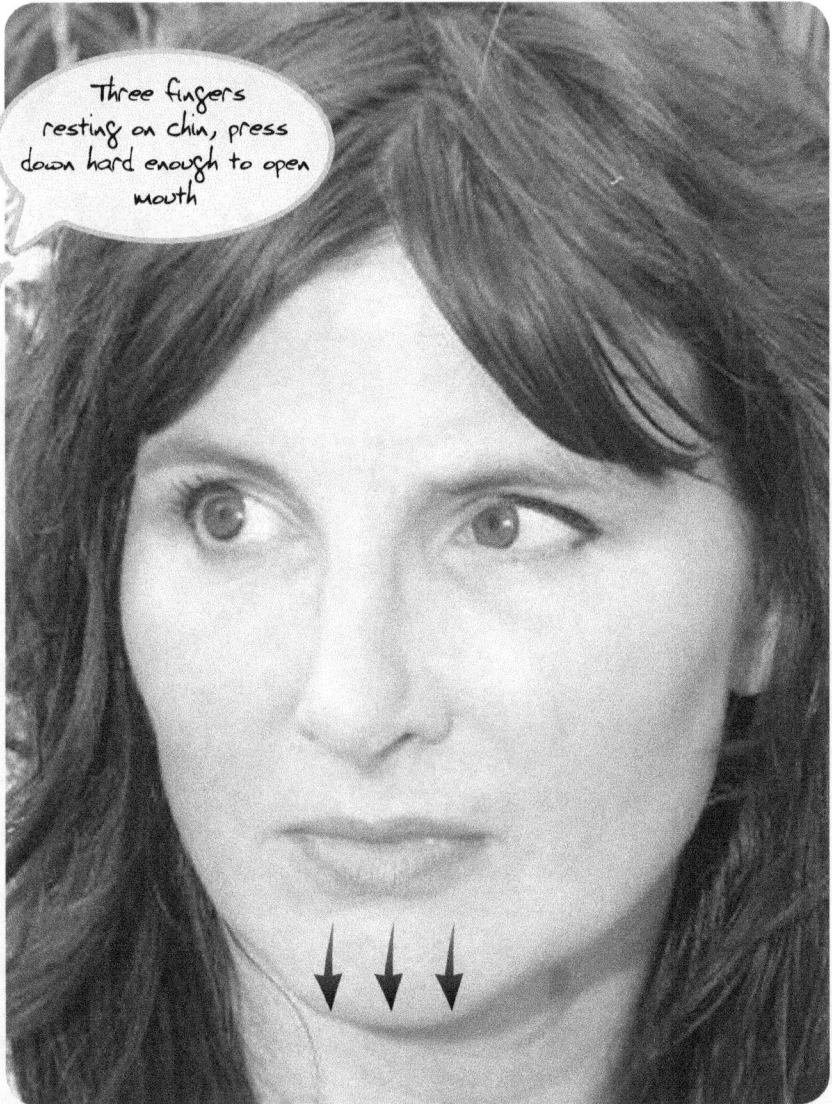

1. Using three fingers of one hand, push down on the jawbone so the mouth opens wide.

2. Slowly bring the lower jaw up until the mouth is closed.

3. Repeat the movement 10 times, counting to four each time.

Checklist

These muscles are skeletal muscles, like the ones in the body. They move a joint (the jaw), and it's important to take care not to damage it, so ask your doctor if you have any doubts about using the jaw, and don't attempt to do extra work for these muscles.

A little of this exercise has a striking effect on the appearance of the face, but more than a little soon makes the face look square and bulky around the jaw.

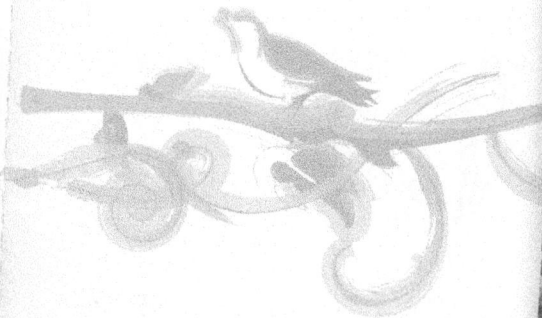

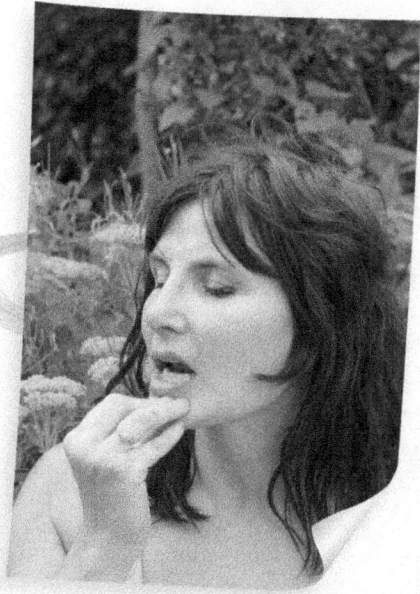

Alternative 4
Nose wrinkle

Type. Minor structural exercise.

Muscle. Angular head of the levator labii.

Result. Lifts flesh either side of the nose vertically.

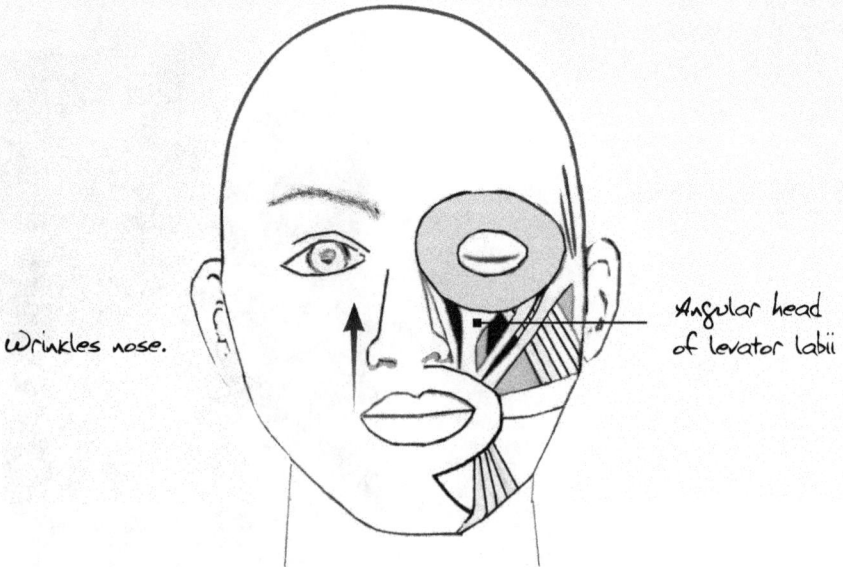

Wrinkles nose.

Angular head
of levator labii

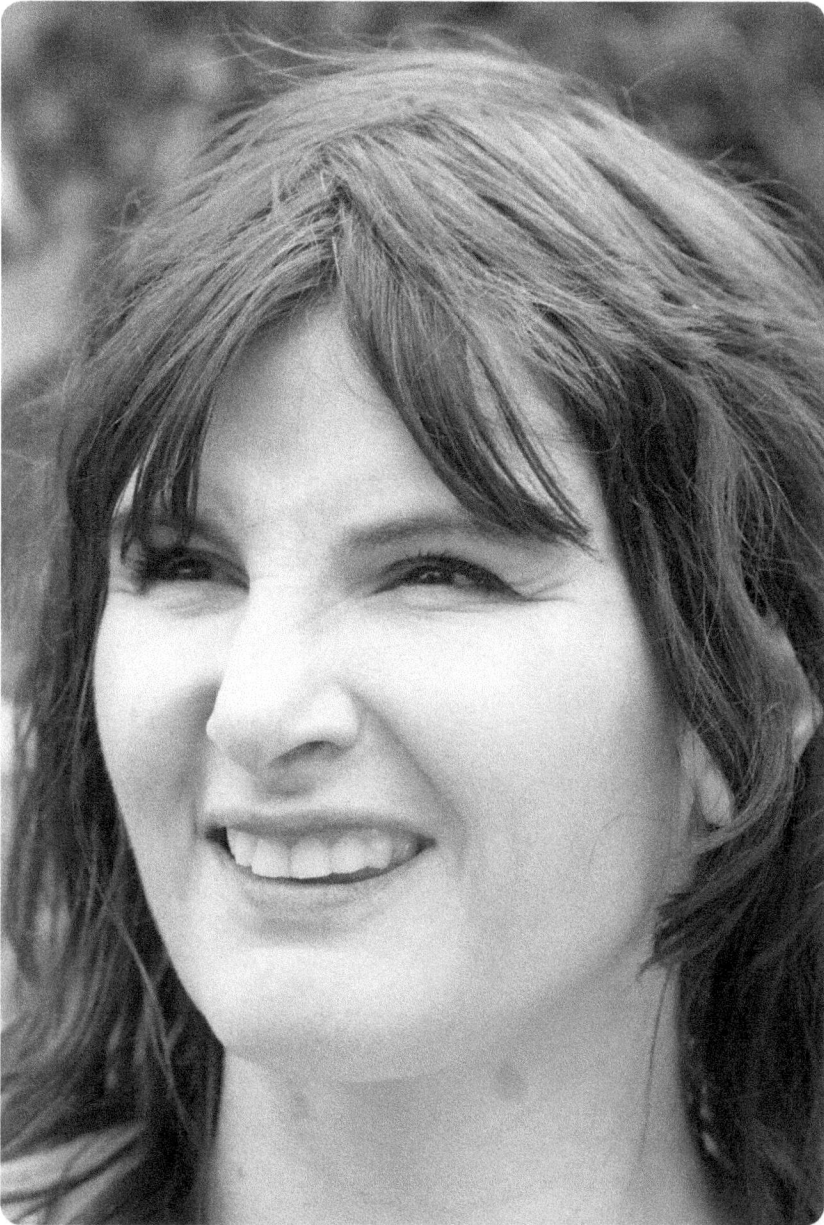

Again, try the movement out to see how it feels before you begin to exercise. The nose wrinkle is fairly straightforward though.

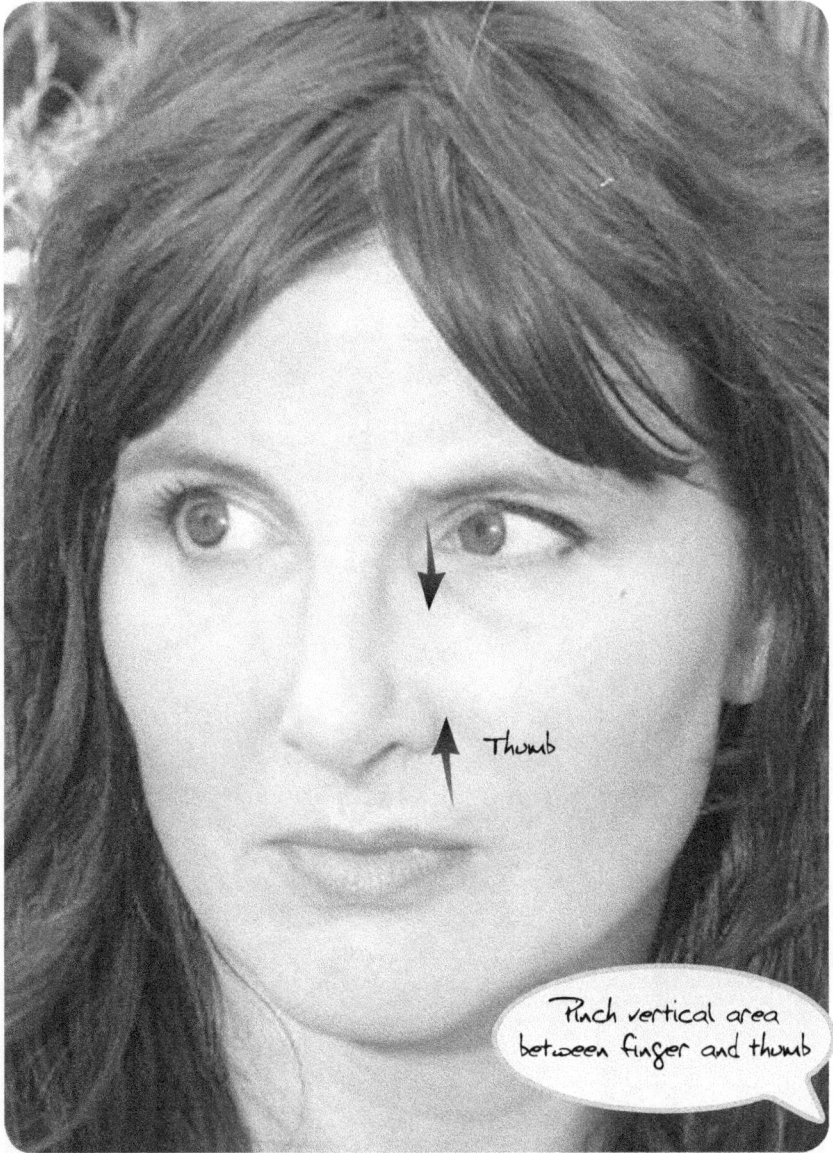

1. Pinch a chunk of flesh horizontally, close to the nose

2. Wrinkle the nose!

3. Repeat 10 times, as quickly as you can.

Checklist

✳ It's much easier to grasp this area if you grasp above and below it rather than trying to grip it in the same way as exercise 1. See the diagram.

✳ It's nice to have the area nicely toned, but building it up isn't really desirable... the muscles that make happy expressions should be stronger than this one so that the cheek curves out at the cheekbone rather than being built-up all the way across.

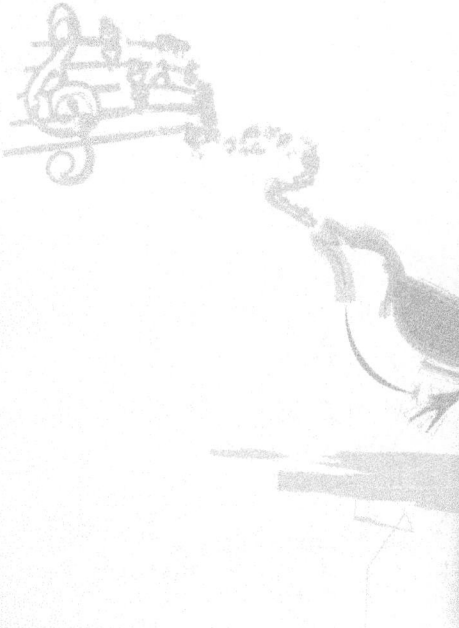

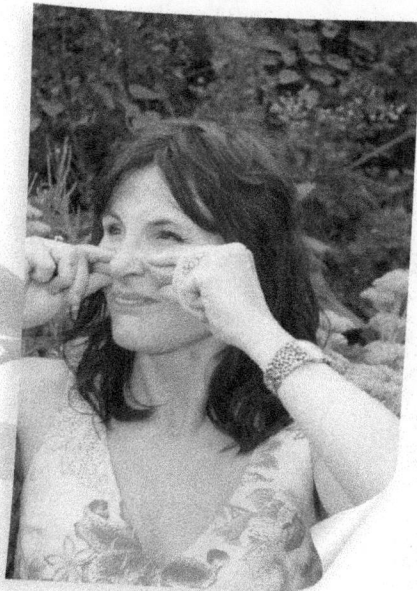

Alternative 5

Lower lip

Type.   Occasional spot-training exercise

Muscle.   Quadratus labii inferioris

Result.   Maintains firmness around lower lip

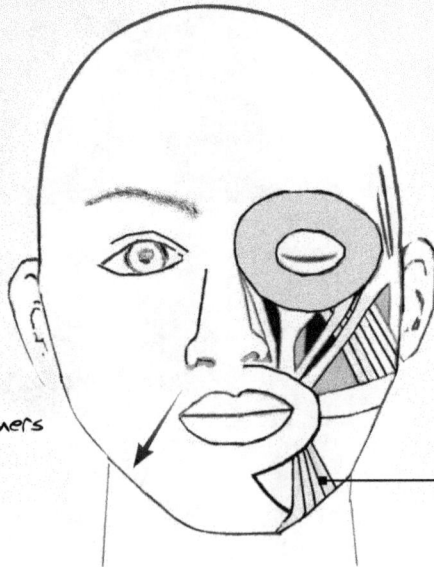

Pulls down corners of lower lip.

Quadratus labii inferioris

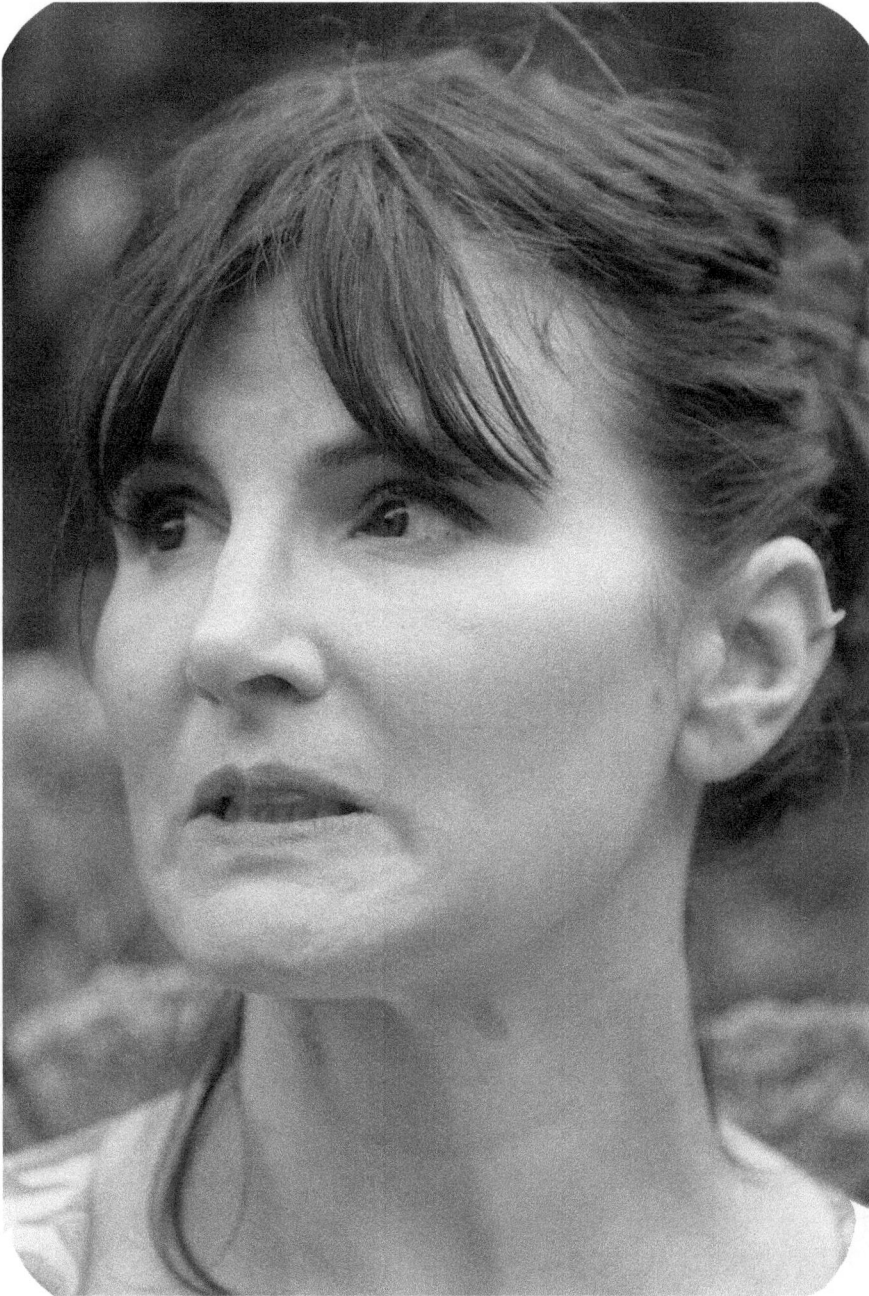

The first time you do the exercise try out the muscle without using hands... the depressor labii pulls the lower lip down and causes it ᴜ out thus. See why we don't exercise this muscle very often.

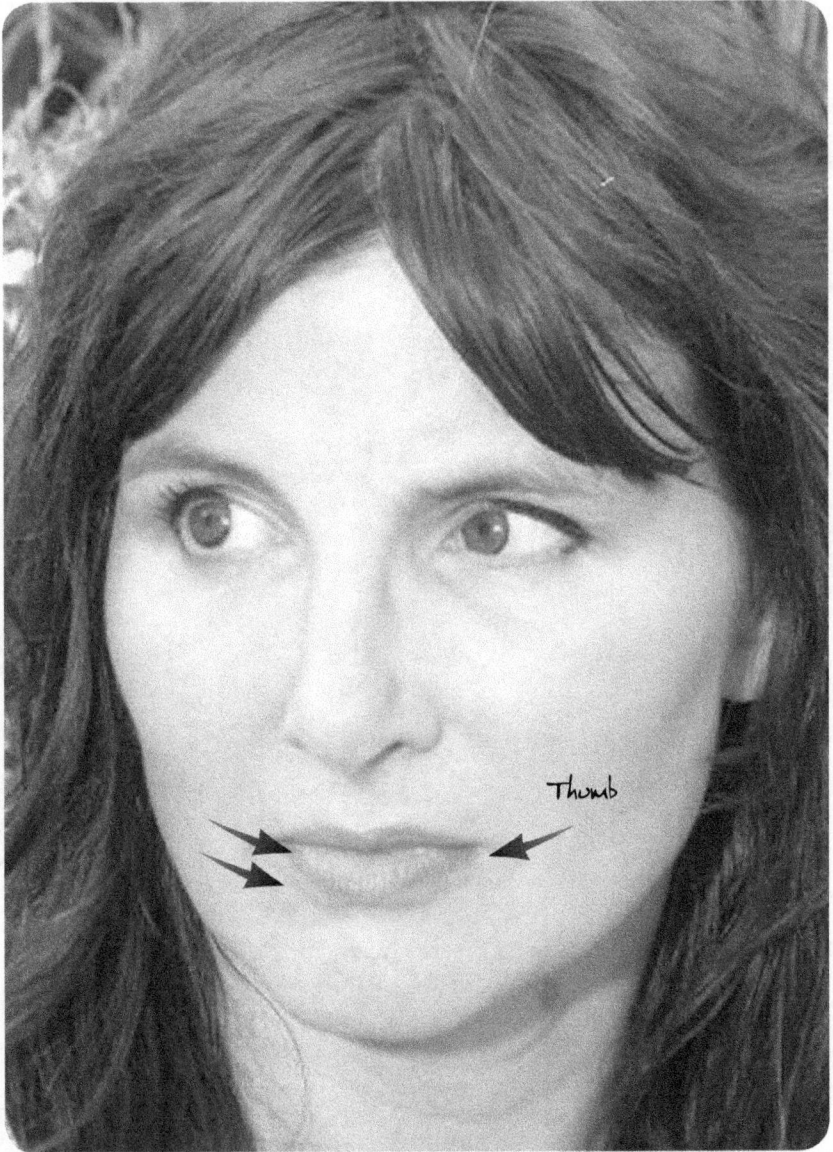

Thumb

1. Pinch the lower lip between fingers and thumb.

2. Try to push your lower lip forward.

3. Repeat 10 times as quickly as you can.

Checklist

* Pinch the largest area of the lower lip you can manage to make it more difficult to perform the exercise, and to increase the stretch.

* Although you don't want to build the lower lip area, work the muscle as thoroughly as you can. It's much simpler to give it the occasional intensive workout than to spend time every day doing little gentle exercises.

* This is just a spot-treatment for the area around the lower lip. It's not desirable to train it to the point where it builds up, but a little work will keep it firm and the skin attached to it smooth.

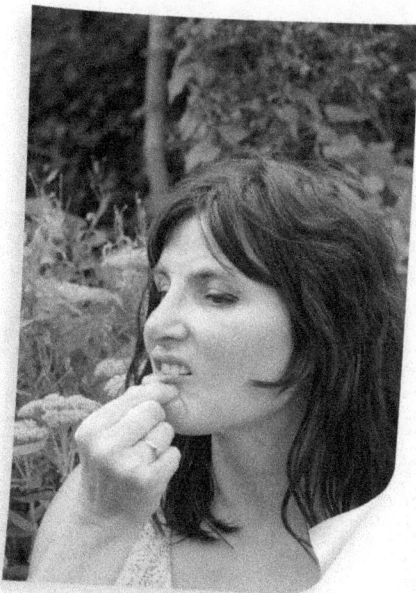

Alternative 6
Chin up

Type.   Minor structural exercise.

Muscle.   Mentalis.

Result.   Lifts the meaty bit of the chin and reverses any elongation there.

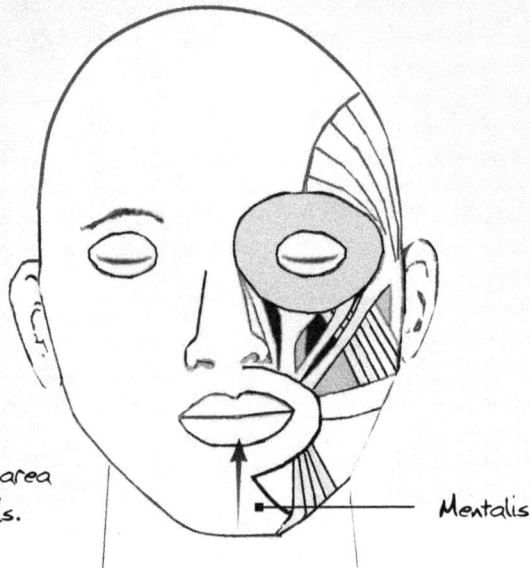

Pulls fleshy area of chin upwards.

Mentalis

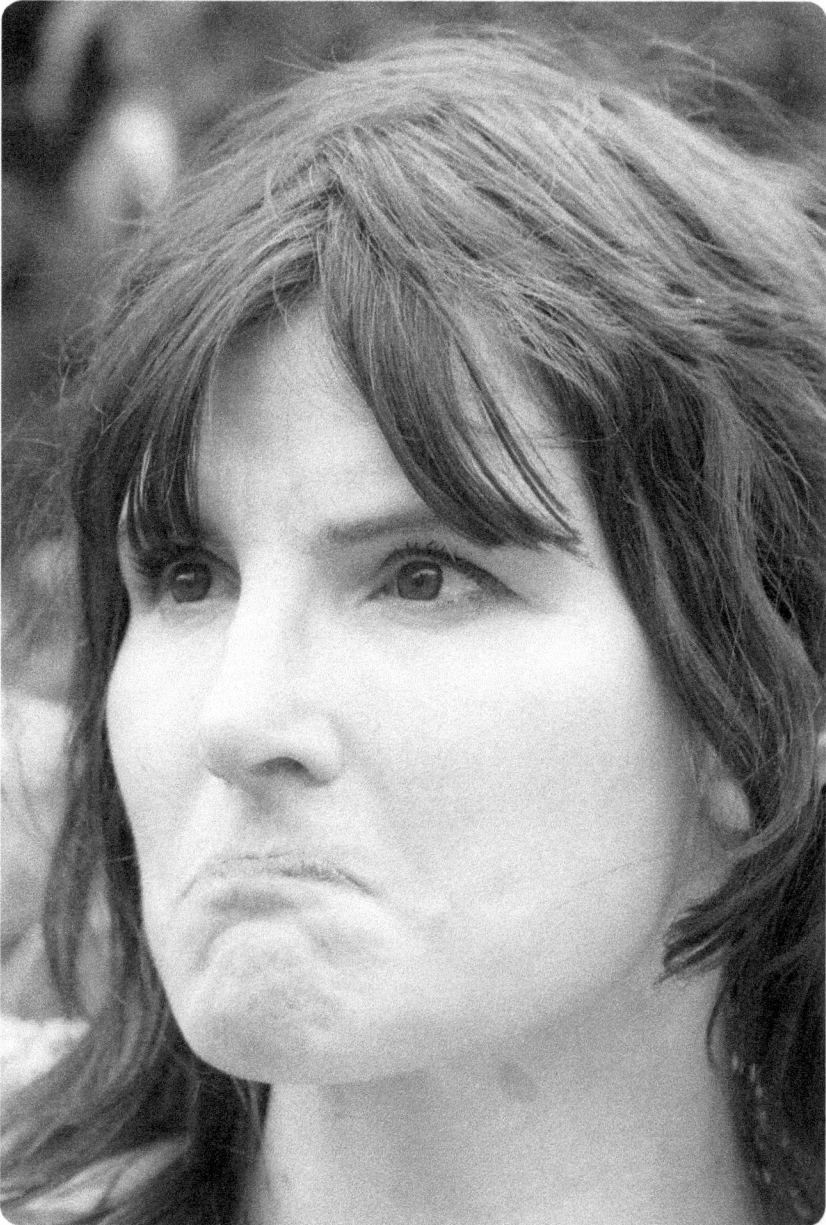

Once again, the first time you do the exercise, try out the muscle without using the hands... mentalis draws the meaty part of the chin up and
causes it to dimple as above. Again we don't want to stick like this.

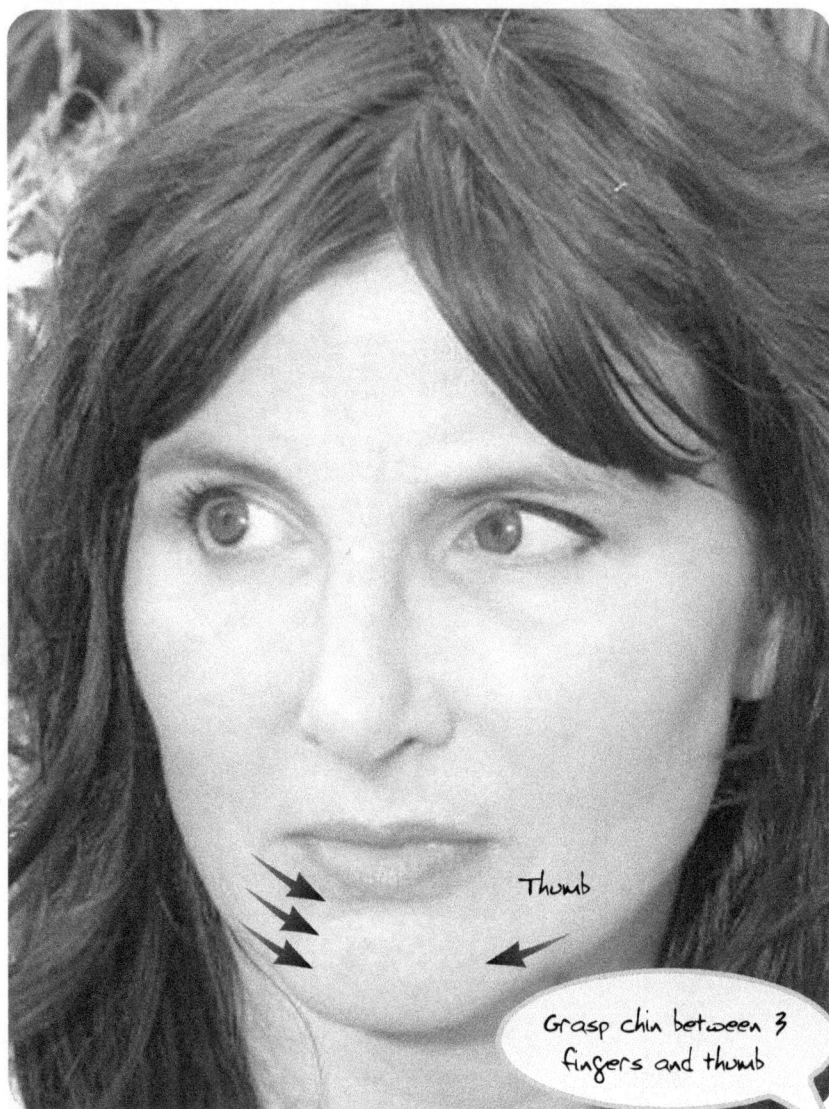

1. Pinch the lower lip between fingers and thumb.

2. Press the lips firmly together, paying special attention to the upward movement of the lower lip.

3. Repeat the movement 10 times as rapidly as you can.

Checklist

* Again it's good to exercise this muscle seldom and intensely rather than frequently and gently.

* This exercise gives a nice little tilt to the meat of the chin that has dropped with gravity and time. However, the mentalis is also the muscle that causes the dimpling effect of many little bumps and dips in the chin, so it's important not to make it too powerful. On the bright side, you should be able to see your chin dimple as you perform this exercise, so it's easy to spot when you're doing it correctly. If not, keep going through the motions until you get it right.

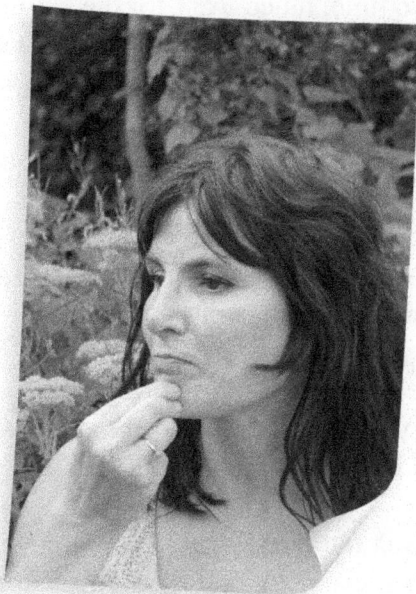

Chapter nine

About firming & thickening skin

Massage (exercise specifically for skin)

To save time, much work for the skin is incorporated into the exercises themselves, but the skin really benefits from any extra work you can do on it. There's no right or wrong way to massage your face, but this is how I do it

Pinch chunks of it, tug it away from the face and do three little tugs at each spot..

Do this everywhere it's possible to tug skin away from the face... along the jawbone, mid and upper cheek, eye area and neck.

Where the skin is too tight against the bone to pull away from the face, for example on the forehead, chin and nose, just pinch and squeeze the area between finger and thumb three times.

This isn't a magic formula... any firm handling of the skin will improve its strength, elasticity and thickness. So rather in the spirit of the exercise diagrams here's a way you could approach handling your face.

The lighter areas of the picture show where you can pull the skin effectively, the darker areas are where you need to pinch it. If you can, do both sides of the face together to save time.

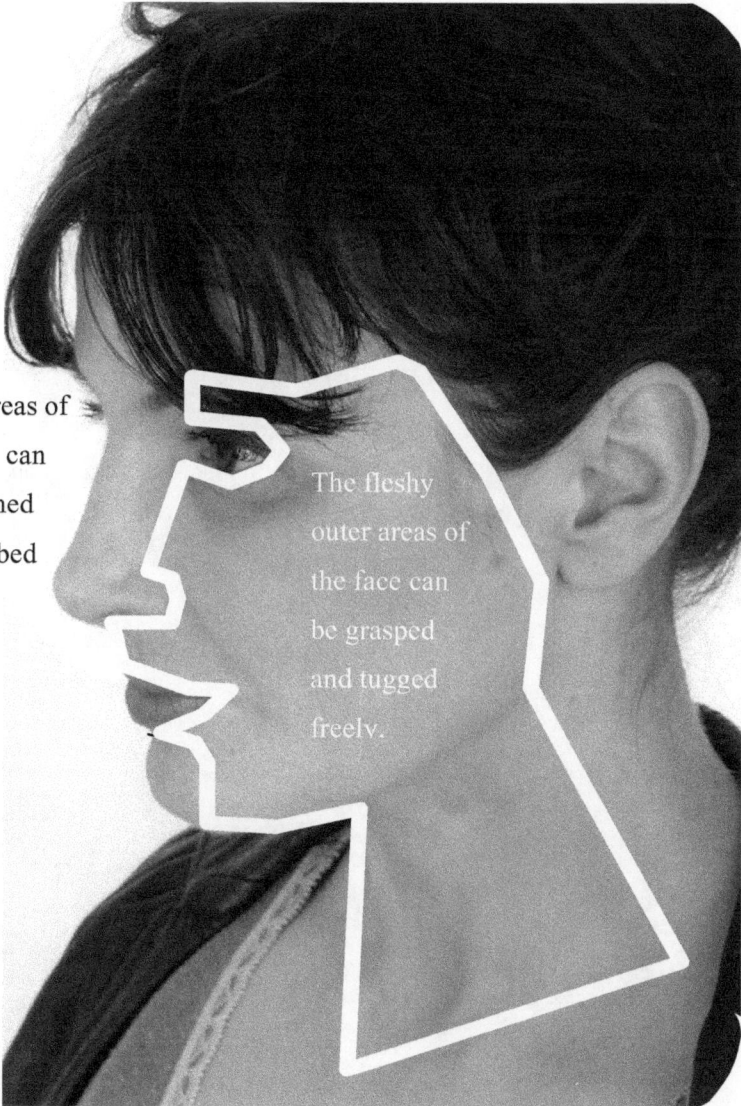

Bony areas of the face can be pinched and rubbed

The fleshy outer areas of the face can be grasped and tugged freely.

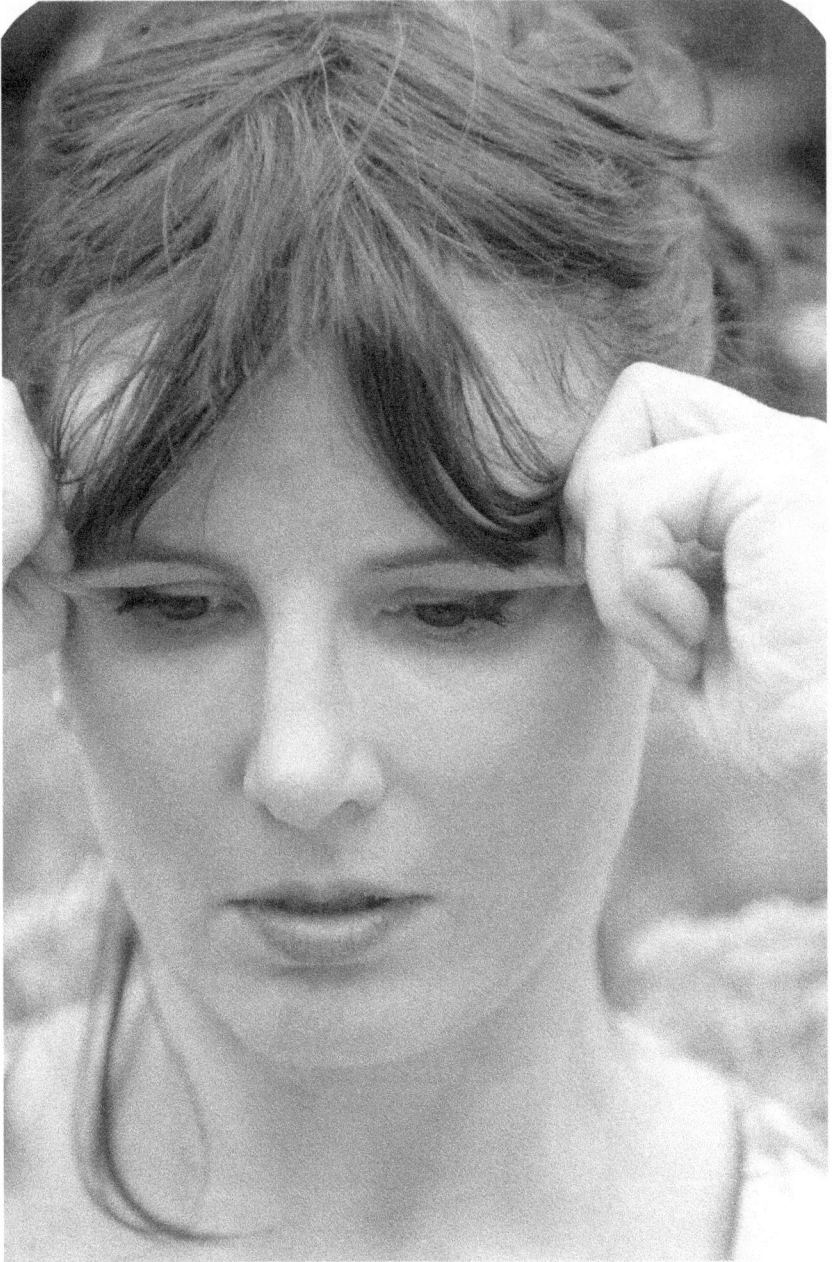

Massaging eyebrows… pull brow tissue away from face, tug and enjoy it.

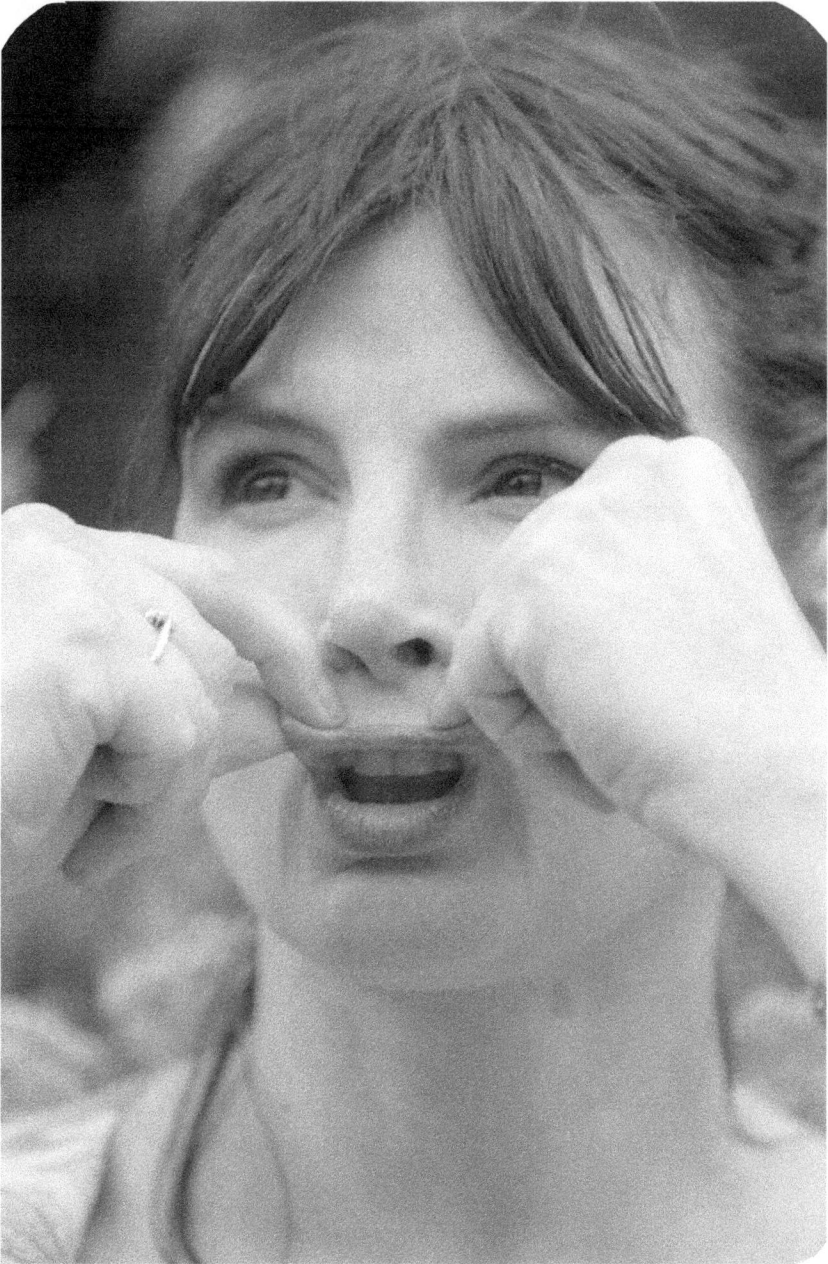

Massage the lip by pulling it firmly.

123

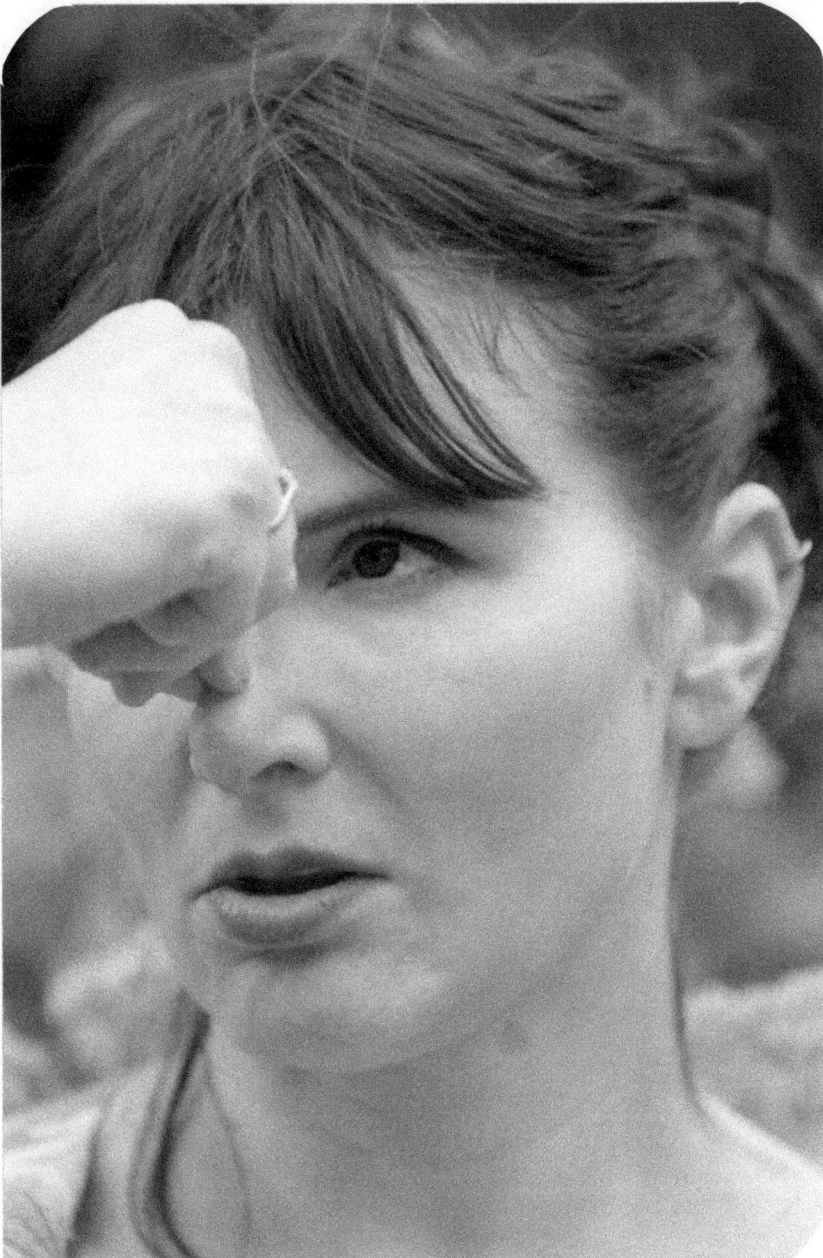

Just nip at tight areas like the nose.

Other ways of challenging your skin

Body brushing works well on the face. Do as often as you like, you only need to spend a few seconds on each area of the face. You can close the eyes and brush over the lids, but be gentle or you might poke your eye with the bristles.

Again, I haven't found it matters much at all which direction you brush in… the idea is to challenge the skin and give it a little spur, so feel free to brush upwards, downwards, left to right or in circles. I'm sure there are advantages to brushing in certain directions, but I don't feel qualified to say what they are. This needs somebody else's book.

Cold water provides another way to challenge the skin. It's effective at least in the short term at making your face feel firmer. This is because the skin itself contains tiny muscles that erect the hairs when you get cold. When they're fully contracted you can see them standing up as goosebumps. How much long-term benefit there is from making them do a little work each day I've no idea. Some women swear that splashing their breasts with cold water every morning keeps them firm, but this is a bit hard to quantify!

It is known that people who spend significant time in cold water retain more body fat than average as they get older, presumably because the body lays down a layer of fat to insulate itself from the cold. Olympic swimmers are a different shape from Olympic track and field athletes or other sports competitors. They have the same muscularity, but the lines of the body are sleeker and the shapes of the muscles is less pronounced: body fat.

For the face this would be fantastic, as fat in the face looks youthful and pretty. It's worth making the face cold a couple of times a day to give the facial fat something to think about.

Chapter ten
How to shine

Being seen again

At some point a woman notices she's become invisible. It's as baffling as it is annoying, and I used to believe it was because your status in society depended on your attractiveness to men. But it isn't that, it's just a misunderstanding that can easily be straightened out.

Notice how you're holding your jaw at the moment. It might be held up and back like it was when you were a young girl, or it might have fallen forward and just be hanging there, probably pulling the rest of the face down with it. We talk about 'letting yourself go' and there does come a time in mid-life where maintaining the poised-for-action muscles of youth just feels like too much effort, and we let it go.

An exaggerated version of the relaxation of the facial muscles is the face a child makes when they pull a 'long face'. They let all their facial muscles sag and the jaw drop. At the same time, to underline the point, the shoulders, chest and arms lose their childish It says very clearly that the child is disinclined to do what's been suggested and finds it a great effort.

By contrast, lifting up the face, wide eyes, high eyebrows, and the chin forward shows eagerness.

I use these extremes to compare the effect given off by a face where the muscles have lengthened to that of a person with good muscle tone. The toned face looks keener and more alert than the older face that looks 'tired'.

I think the people who pass over us respect us every bit as much as they respect the next person, they just aren't registering us because other people's faces are giving out more obvious signals. Other people are signalling more strongly that they're ready or that it's their turn.

126

From very early in your training, the muscles reawaken and you hold the face differently, looking ready to engage with whatever the encounter might be about, subtly giving off the signal that you're about to speak, smile, do something that people should attend to, and one day you, to your amazement, you become visible again.

Understanding how to hold the face

This has been called 'facial posture'. Just as athletes and dancers carry themselves nicely, the way someone holds their face is key to how they look. At the beginning of your training it probably seems like really hard work to hold your chin up and turn up the corners of the mouth, but after a while it becomes second nature. Athletes aren't conscious of standing erect or of holding the abdominal muscles in, and they aren't tense as they do so. Letting the stomach hang out and the shoulders slump isn't really relaxation, is it.

Holding your face in a good way soon becomes effortless as your muscles regain their tonus, but it's encouraging to consider what you're working towards.

There are many examples of older women whose body language exudes presence. Margot Fonteyn thrilled the world during her 40s and 50s when she danced with Rudolph Nureyev. Mae West's distinctive stance and walk (copied from a female impersonator) didn't appear on film until she was in her 40s. Shirley Bassey's dramatic gestures and poses still work for her aged 80.... There are few people less invisible; because they strongly project certain aspects of their personality in the way they use their bodies.

Holding the head nicely has three advantages. On the one hand you command more attention, on the other you look prettier. Almost any expression looks better than exhaustion.

The third aspect to facial posture is its connection with emotional health. We've learned through a number of experiments dating back to the seventies that facial expression creates moods as well as reflecting them.

Smiling constantly makes other people uncomfortable, especially in the UK where we have a deep suspicion of smiling people. But in the course of your training you'll learn which muscles are engaged when you feel happy, alert or confident. You can focus on these without actually making the full-blown expression, so that you communicate the appropriate emotion to others and induce it in yourself.

Other signals of alertness include holding the brows in a slightly lifted position and open eyes, the same features that we find attractive, naturally. But the jaw is key. Exercising the temple and jaw-angle chewing muscles pulls the back of the jaw as high as a young girl's.

When you have thought of yourself as faded and learned to accept your place on the sidelines, the idea of stepping into the light sounds a bit daunting. But it's not about how loudly you proclaim your presence; it's about learning to share your authentic qualities with other people rather than burying them inside you.

At some points in your life your face can look wonderful in a way nobody on earth can imitate. That's what you can achieve with this book. Instead of striving to reconstruct yourself as something you're not, you can enjoy everything you are.

I am incomparable

It's the purpose of advertisers to bring about a condition of dissatisfaction and lack: you have to feel as though you're missing something so that you'll feel the need to buy whatever it is they are selling. The images, especially those of people, are unrealistic so that the need is never satisfied; this is their job.

We're not as happy as we could be because we accept its values and its slogans. Looking through a fashion magazine is a demoralising experience not just because the model is physically perfect, but because the figure is always at a remove from the reader, ignoring you, looking at you with cool disregard or blatantly pouting at your boyfriend. Even if you have a face and body just like them you have no answer to the series of alpha females who are deliberately posed as though you were nothing, and you feel put in your place over and over again.

In fact nobody is more beautiful than you are. If you look at a room full of children you might see that one has prettier hair or straighter teeth than another, but every one of them is lovely to look at, and their facial quirks add to their charm. But there comes a point in their lives where their faces will be judged and compared instead of appreciated and enjoyed.

The media have told us that we want to see a certain type of woman, young, slim and flawless, but I'd suggest that actually there's nothing inherently more attractive about this type than any other.

In the 1980s I used to train with weights and read just about anything I could find about the subject. There was no Internet a few books and especially magazines, many of which were glossy, expensive affairs packed with advertisements for supplements, of which there were a great number. The rest of the pages were taken up with hugely muscular people who were promoting the goods alongside their training routines. In the photo-shoots the women were dressed glamorously and posed as though they were highly desirable. At first these women looked strange and very unattractive indeed, but after a few weeks of being exposed to the pictures I began to feel rather small and underdeveloped, and the bodies in fashion magazines began to look incredibly thin.

The way the world is presented to us makes a huge difference to what we aspire to. We hear the words of advertising and publicity, good, lovely, clean, pretty, amazing, best, beautiful, fantastic, and apply them to what's put in front of us. The bodybuilding magazines replace one ideal with another, albeit a more robust, well-nourished one, but you can take the language of beauty, disregard the thought of perfection and carry it easily into your daily life.
Believe it or not, this language is available to anyone, and is not bound to the narrow vision of what MTV and Hollywood are giving us. For a long time we've hesitated to use the words except in the context of the idealised images

created for us by a team of experts. The words belong out there with in an idealised world, not for us. But they deserve to mean something enduring and interesting instead of being dumbed down to mean something so obvious and trivial. We get into the habit of thinking everything must be there at once and on the surface and grab your attention, but if you begin to use this vocabulary for yourself when you see your friends or your garden, you can put their appealing qualities in their rightful place. It's good to look for what's of real value in your world, so that at least one person is using their own vision and imagination. It's the world of the media that's inadequate, not yours.

This is partly why, as you will see, you're asked to tell yourself you are beautiful and elegant and radiant when you're training. You may think this is a bit silly, but it can't hurt to speak to yourself with a little affection and respect, and counting is not so exciting that you can't replace it with something different.

Training your face and handling your skin feels good, so it automatically makes you feel happier with what you have and gives you a powerful connection with what is alive and real. This should help give you the confidence to listen to your own voice, and to look at other people's faces with admiration and respect, without needing to compare or measure yourself against them. Once you accept other faces, it's easy to accept your own.

Your face is good enough... just as a body of any shape looks lovely when its muscles are firm and it moves easily, the face will do the same.

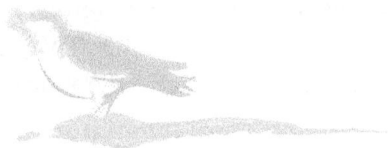

Appendix one
Frequently asked questions

1. I'm afraid to pull my face.

Don't be Just take the plunge and you'll be astonished at the results. If you read the first chapter of this book I hope it will persuade you how much you gain by taking a bold approach.

2. Why aren't there any exercises for under the eyes?

There are! The eye muscle is circular... it goes right round the eye, including beneath it. Although you're holding the flesh at the side of the eye during The Wish exercise the entire muscle is worked equally. Wish is a great exercise for under the eyes.

3. Why aren't there many exercises for the lower face?

This is intentional, and it's because there's no advantage to building the lower face, as any loss of firmness in the lower face isn't caused by deterioration of these muscles, but by the upper face losing tone and sliding down so that the lower face looks sagging and fatty.

131

Building the lower face muscles does nothing to lift the face, it merely bulks up the area around the jaw and lower face. It's the upper face muscles that can reverse the effects of gravity. draw the sagging areas of the lower face upwards to reveal the jawline and lower face that have been obscured by the downward shift of flesh over time. There's sufficient material in the 'occasional' section to keep the lower face firm.

I apologise, but from here the faqs seem to have lost their question element. Still, I hope the following addresses some of the things that people would like to know about.

4. Temporary wrinkles

When things aren't going smoothly, people report some or all of the side-effects described in this chapter. First, the facialista may notice the development of temporary wrinkles around the eyes and mouth. These are caused by the facial muscles not relaxing completely after exercise. The skin is entirely bonded to the muscle... if the muscle is at all misshapen, the skin gets skewed into wrinkles. The easiest way to explain why they might be more apparent early on in your training is to imagine a piece of foam or sponge with a piece of cloth bonded to it on one side

If it's squeezed with the hands a new piece of foam automatically regains its original shape, but over the years there comes a point where the process becomes slow, the sponge begins to look a bit lumpy and eventually the sponge won't go back to its original shape at all. At this point the bonded fabric has wrinkled to accommodate the uneven surface. The deep lines on the face aren't caused by creasing the skin, they're caused by the uneven muscle not allowing the skin to lie flat

So there are two methods we could use to address the problem of the shapeless sponge. One is to stop squeezing it altogether, in which case it will gradually allow itself to return to its original dimensions. Many people do the exact same thing for their faces by getting muscle-paralysing injections (Botox).

The other way to revive the shape of the worn sponge is to replace it with a new one! This is what we do, by producing stronger, healthier and more youthful muscle cells that provide a smooth, youthful surface for the skin cells to lie on. But it's not possible to go out and buy a new facial structure, you have to gradually phase one musculature out as the new cells form so a certain number of our muscles will be the older ones for a time.

The process of building new muscle means using that muscle, squeezing the sponge hard. In the time after an exercise session you might well see wrinkling produced because the old muscle has retained the shape of the facial exercise..and pulled the skin with it. It's nothing to worry about at all, because once all the new cells have formed, the muscle will be very elastic, strong and reluctant to leave an imprint.. The puckered muscle will flatten out over the time till the next exercise session .

If you were to go to the gym and work hard your shoulders or leg may be stiff for a day or two. You'd understand it was the body's immediate response to the exercise, not a permanent state of affairs because you have ruined your leg muscles. Temporary wrinkling is just like that, it's the body's immediate response to the exercise, not an indication of how your muscles are developing.

In all the cases In this chapter, I'd have the same recommendation. You can either live with it secure in the knowledge that the phase will pass. Or you could stop training and completely rest your face until it goes away.

Either way, it's very important to enjoy your face, not to scrutinise it for imperfections . The aim is to love your face. There's a temptation to look too closely, to be impatient for progress like a dieter constantly consulting their scales. I would love it if people would forget about the mirror and enjoy their faces.

5. Puffy areas

These are the little puffy bits either side of your mouth. They are truly not as noticeable as you think, and if they feel firm and knotty, then like temporary wrinkling and hollow cheeks, they are usually a response to the action of the muscles when you exercise, like the muscles bunching after you work out in the gym. They don't stay like that forever, and they're not really developing into bunched shapes, they're just forming the shapes they make when they're flexed hard.

Again, if you wanted, you could take a very slow approach to shaping your face, that is, just exercise once every fortnight and the rest of the time concentrate on pulling the skin and giving it a nice stretch. Or you could rest until the pouches flatten out, in order to reassure yourself that they will, then carry on in the knowledge that if you leave plenty of time before an event you want to look great for, you can let your face unscrunch and depuff into looking really fab.

Occasionally they are a skin issue. These areas can also be slow to firm and lift, and the firmer flesh around them makes them look quite pouchy. The skin can be considerably slower to respond to than the muscle. For more detail, please see the post on the skin (7 in this section)

I don't for a minute mean to trivialise people's concerns with this. The following suggestions are intended to encourage and cheer you up, not to dismiss something that you are conscious of.

i. It's worth noting that the area looks less smooth and refined when you're not feeling happy with your face. Over time, as the muscles go stronger and carry the face effortlessly, its expression changes, the corners of the mouth lift. If you give yourself the hint of a smile in the mirror everything becomes smooth and rounded.

ii. When other people look at us they look at our eyes and lips. When someone looks in the mirror the focus is entirely different, and it's easy to lose sight of all the beauty in a face, by shining a light so intensely on the elements that we're not at peace with.

6. Hollow cheeks

This is another side-effect that affects some people . The buccinators (large cheek muscle) pull the cheek in against the back teeth, and after a few training sessions it trains it to do this very effectively. Once again this is a response to the training itself rather than anything to do with the way the muscles are developing. The muscles of the cheeks are growing thicker through the exercise, but they retain the pulled-in shape of the exercise after a session, and can look as though they have shrunk and taken all the fat out of your face. And once again, the solution is to take a long rest, just keep resting till your face returns to normal, when you'll be able to see how your cheeks really have developed. People vary a great deal both in the rate of developing the musculature of their face, and in the rate at which the side-effects of an exercise session might last. But everyone can succeed with patience... this means being willing to rest and allow your face to recover as much as doing the exercises . I'd suggest to anyone who would like a serene progression towards a more lifted, more radiant face to train one month, rest one month.

7. Areas of less-firm skin.

The skin reacts very quickly to being overtrained by becoming less elastic and less healthy-looking. It can be quickly and easily revived by taking a few days off and allowing the fibres that have been broken down by the exercise to repair themselves and produce fresh, resilient skin cells in their place.

Over the longer term, the skin may not keep pace with the alteration in the muscle shape. Handling it and massaging it helps massively, but the places on the skin where the skin is not bonded to the muscle need time to adapt to the new, more compact and lifted shape. The main area that this concerns is the neck, although even here the muscle's attachment to the skin on the lower part of the face pulls the rest of the skin upwards to an extent. It will adapt... even the abundance of skin produced in pregnancy eventually conforms to the flatter stomach after the baby is born. It may never become perfect (mine certainly hasn't),but over time it will grow significantly tighter than it was straight after the birth. The skin adapts itself to the shape it covers all by itself, without the need for special creams, or even massage. If you choose to devote some time to pulling the skin, especially in the neck, and also in the puffy-mouth area, where the stack of muscles cross each other, just before the place where they merge with the skin, your skin will follow the natural course of things and conform to the new, compact shape even more success-fully.

8. I don't look any different!

First thing is to consider whether you're performing the exercises correctly... they are simple to do, but it's possible to make two mistakes that make them much less effective.

i. Be sure to use the correct muscle. Actually, even partly using it will do. It's quite simple with the Day 1 exercises as the muscles are all pulling the mouth outwards. If your lip is moving away from the centre rather than pursing or puckering the lips you're on the right track, and even if you're not sure which exact muscle you're using, you soon will, and for now you're performing the exercise accurately enough to start seeing results, so that isn't the reason you don't seem to be getting anywhere!

Just to add, the precise place where you grip the chunk of flesh isn't impor-tant at all. Almost any chunk of flesh will do the trick, the muscle has to work harder because the flesh-grip tightens the skin, restricting the amount of 'give' in it, making it more difficult to move it. So whatever you're doing chunk-of-flesh-wise matters very little, it's the direction of the movement you need to concentrate on. To repeat, you should be pulling outwards toward the hairline, preferably towards the area (eg temple, eye) indicated in the exercise you're doing.

ii. Range of movement. The other thing I may not have made clear enough in the book is the importance of not gripping too tightly. You need to be able to move the muscle till it's fully clenched, not grasp it so hard that you can't move it at all and perform the equivalent of trying to lift a weight that's too heavy for you and just straining against it. The hands will be relaxed enough

136

to loosen your grip and be pulled open as the muscle bunches the `chunk of flesh.

Bearing all this in mind, if you're still not getting the results you were hoping for, you need to tighten your grip so that the muscle works hard (but is able to move through its full range of motion- see above!), and maybe step up your repetitions to 25 for a week or so.

You have almost certainly made progress, it's just that sometimes the skin needs time to adapt and is masking the lovely structure you have created underneath. Sometimes changes happen in bursts of growth followed by periods where everything seems to remain the same.

9. Taking it slowly, which comes up in all the above.

I lifted my face with a form of stop-start training, always doing fewer exercises than recommended, training very hard for a few days, then stopping because something else caught my attention. I cut out on exercises rather than adding more, and for a very long time I've exercised only the muscles in this book. It made for a peaceful journey, although that wasn't intentional. If my face had a trace of gauntness or loss of softness I stopped training until it went. At one point I had wrinkles around my eyes, but everything else looked better, and then they went too. It took me until a couple of years ago to figure out why they appeared and why they went. The way to avoid side-effects is to take your time, and not be in a rush to get your new face.

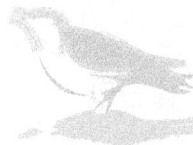

Appendix two
Contacts

Louise Annette

http://www.agelessifwedare.com/
http://louiseannette.proboards.com/index.cgi

Photography

Sabel Carrillo

0778 996 3783
33 Cowley Rd, Oxford OX4 1HP
sabel@studioblanco.co.uk

Claire Williams

07765 240 066
info@clairewilliamsphotography.co.uk

Graphic Design

Michael Ward

07702 101 690
mikeward@me.com

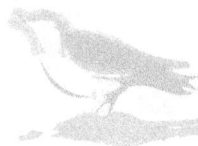